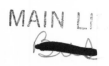

ALLEN COUNTY PUBLIC LIBRARY

FORT WAYNE, INDIANA 46802

You may return this book to any agency, branch,
or bookmobile of the Allen County Public Library.

DEMCO

FUTURE
VISION

FUTURE VISION

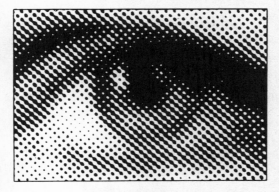

SPACE-AGE TECHNIQUES TO SAVE YOUR SIGHT

**ROBERT H. RUBMAN, M.D.
& HOWARD ROTHMAN**
Illustrated by John M. Thompson

DODD, MEAD & COMPANY
NEW YORK

Copyright © 1987 by Lewis A. Goodman

All illustrations © 1987, Medical Marketing Associates, Jackson Hole, Wyoming

A GAMUT BOOK

Published by Dodd, Mead & Company, Inc.

71 Fifth Avenue, New York, N.Y. 10003

Distributed in Canada by

McClelland and Stewart Limited, Toronto

Manufactured in the United States of America
Designed by Joyce Levatino

First Edition

1 2 3 4 5 6 7 8 9 10

Future Vision has been packaged for Dodd, Mead & Company by
Lewis A. Goodman

Library of Congress Cataloging-in-Publication Data

Rubman, Robert H.
Future vision.

Bibliography: p.
Includes index.
1. Eye—Surgery. 2. Ophthalmology—Popular works.
I. Rothman, Howard. II. Title.
RE80.R83 1987   617.7'1   87-5238
ISBN 0-396-08892-9
ISBN 0-396-08956-9 {PBK.}

Contents

Introduction

In today's society, vision is usually considered to be our most important sense. Many people certainly live happy and productive lives without it, but those of us who are blessed with good eyesight probably would not trade it for all the money in the world. We use it for practically every activity other than sleep. We rely on it so heavily, in fact, that we generally expect it to serve us well until the day we die.

Despite its importance, however, things do go wrong. Vision dims and blurs for no apparent reason. Closeup or faraway objects may be hard to see clearly. The aging process—and our increasing lifespan—can take its toll. Diseases like diabetes and hypertension will affect our eyes. Accidents and illnesses may destroy our vision.

Although eyesight has remained one of life's most puzzling mysteries—no one has ever been able to develop a universally accepted explanation for its everyday workings—a number of exciting advances have offered new hope to those of us who suffer from various vision impairments. Medical doctors who specialize in eye treatment have discovered more and more about certain common eye disorders in recent years, while a simultaneous technological sophistication has enabled them to develop space-age treatments for many of these once untreatable vision problems.

As recently as World War II, however, these physicians—known as *ophthalmologists*—were severely hampered by the crude technology and primitive techniques that were then available to them. Although their medical field actually existed for hundreds of years, the practice of eye surgery had advanced with excruciating slowness because the tools and techniques that were necessary for such intricate procedures evolved little, if at all, since their initial introduction many generations before.

The postwar invention of the operating microscope—particularly the giant leaps forward in microsurgery for which this instrument paved the way—finally allowed the field of ophthalmology to enter the twentieth century. Additional developments consistently built upon ophthalmology's ever-growing body of knowledge about the eye and vision, and the revolution in eye care has continued ever since at a rapidly accelerating pace. Many of the procedures that are now considered standard, in fact, actually did not exist even ten years ago.

From the patient's point of view, this eye-care revolution has been responsible for many dramatic changes. It has opened up a variety of new and exciting treatment options, for example, while at the same time improving the safety and effectiveness of most of the ophthalmic surgical methods that are in widespread use today.

In the 1980s, a well-informed patient who is facing eye surgery can insist that the most up-to-date ophthalmic procedures available be performed in a state-of-the-art surgical facility. And in many cases he can also request that the surgery be performed on an outpatient basis—thus allowing him to return home only hours after the operation has been completed instead of remaining in a hospital for three or four days as such surgery routinely required in the past.

While today's high-tech ophthalmic techniques have not totally eliminated the pain and discomfort that once was universally associated with these and other surgical procedures, they *have* drastically reduced the unpleasant side effects common to the majority of medical operations. In the past, most forms of eye surgery involved a rather large incision that, in effect, was created by poking a needle into the patient's eye. Today, the use of space-age instruments like the laser has permitted the surgeon to perform many of these same procedures without making any incision at all. And other procedures, such as cataract removal, involve only an extremely tiny incision.

Pain, of course, is a subjective emotional sensation that is perceived differently by different people who undergo a similar physical experience. Some patients may therefore feel that today's cataract extraction methods are entirely painless, some may report a slight amount of discomfort, and others may complain of moderate pain that requires aspirin or even a mild painkiller to alleviate. In general, however, it is acknowledged that most of today's space-age ophthalmic surgical procedures are relatively pain-free. And additional improvements in technique and technology will continually improve that aspect of eye care as well as many others.

Future Vision is designed specifically for a general public that may still be unaware of the majority of these promising new ophthalmic procedures. It provides vital information for the more than 100 million Americans who wear prescription lenses and the over 11 million Americans who suffer from some type of vision impairment. It offers welcome news for everyone from the senior citizen who no longer is able to read or drive because of a cataract to the nearsighted young adult who is uncomfortable or dissatisfied with corrective lenses.

Future Vision is, however, vastly different from the many other books about eye care that are currently on the market. This is because eye care, unlike diet or exercise or beauty, is not something that can be undertaken solely by the individual.

The space-age solutions that are offered for the various vision problems discussed in this book must be performed by an ophthalmologist, the only medical doctor that specializes in eye care. Rather than offering ways for readers to solve their own vision problems, then, this book helps them to recognize the nature of those problems and then shows them how to find the most up-to-date solution that is available.

But eye care today is marked by more than high-tech tools and techniques—it is marked by *choices.* The patient can choose when it is time to have his cataract removed. He can choose to undergo a surgical alternative to eyeglasses or contact lenses. He can choose to have glaucoma or certain retinal disorders treated by laser surgery. He can choose to have his operation in an outpatient facility. He can even choose to find a new ophthalmologist if he dislikes the method of treatment that his current one suggests.

By clearly and candidly discussing the options that are now available, *Future Vision* will help readers to discover the exciting new tools and techniques that could improve their vision dramatically and forever. In doing so, it answers these and many other questions:

- How does the eye work, and what types of things can go wrong with it?
- How effectively do the new *refractive surgery* procedures improve nearsightedness, farsightedness, and astigmatism in patients who previously relied on prescription eyeglasses or contact lenses?
- What does painless laser surgery mean to those with glaucoma, a leading cause of blindness that is almost always preventable when diagnosed early?
- In these times of decreasing Medicare reimbursement, is outpatient cataract surgery a viable alternative to an expensive hospital stay?
- How can a disease like macular degeneration—which causes a loss of sharp central vision and accompanies the normal aging process—now be eased by laser treatment?
- Can a plastic intraocular lens, an implanted substitute that acts as a built-in contact lens, help the former cataract sufferer to see clearly again?

- In what way can lasers be used to treat retinal tears, which are often indicated by the sudden onset of so-called "flashes" or "floaters" in one eye?
- How often should a forty-year-old obtain a complete eye examination? How about a twenty-year-old? A sixty-year-old?
- How can you discover if your insurance coverage—either private or Medicare—will fund these new high-tech procedures, and how can you submit claims and ask questions?
- Where can you find an eye doctor with the skill and equipment to perform these sight-saving miracles, and how can you be sure that he is the right physician for you?
- What do terms like *YAG laser* and *cryolathe* mean, and how can they be used to treat common vision ailments?
- How are space-age ophthalmologists trained, and what are their feelings about the new procedures?
- Can postoperative cataract patients see as well as they did in their youth?

If you are one of the millions who suffer from a vision problem and would like to save your sight, *Future Vision* can help.

FUTURE VISION

1

The New Ophthalmology

While most of the children born during the last quarter of the twentieth century probably will believe that life has always been a nonstop whirlwind of high-tech inventions and scientific advancements, those of us who predate the marvels of the 1980s know better. We remember a time when air travel was open only to a select few, when televisions and telephones were considered a luxury for the very rich, and when space flights were the exclusive domain of Saturday afternoon serials and speculative science fiction authors.

Today, of course, all this has changed. Parents and their children casually pile onto packed airplanes to embark on regular cross-country visits and globe-trotting vacations. Televisions, often with color and stereophonic sound, glow from nearly every room in our homes. Telephones that record important numbers and then automatically dial them are found in our backyards and even in our cars. As for space travel, once the moon was conquered, what other feat was left to suprise us?

Despite the rapid succession of technological advances that have defined our recent decades, the inventions that actually were responsible for them often came about many years earlier, because it regularly takes quite some time before they fulfill their initial promise. Important inventions usually have served only as stepping stones for further, more far-reaching advances. Ironically, many critically important inventions gain popular acceptance only when society can finally take them for granted.

The same scenario is often repeated in the field of medicine, where technology and technique are combined—usually years apart—to create a miracle that eventually becomes the accepted norm. Few of us wonder any longer about penicillin, for example, even though this critical antibiotic was only discovered in 1929 and first used practically in 1941. And even something as dramatic as a human heart transplant, first performed as recently as 1967, is eventually accepted and replaced in the news by the next remarkable medical development that comes along. Amazing advances like these continue at a mind-boggling pace, too, and nearly every field of medicine is regularly touched by them.

OPHTHALMOLOGY HAS BENEFITED GREATLY FROM THE EXPLOSION IN MEDICAL TECHNOLOGY

Ophthalmology—the branch of medical science that is concerned with the structure, functions, and diseases of the eye—is the one medical field that actually may have achieved the greatest boon from this explosive proliferation of scientific technique and high technology. Although the science had existed for many centuries, a lack of precision tools and precise procedures, coupled with a widespread but understandable willingness to accept the status quo, prohibited many giant steps forward. A recent series of exciting space-age advances, however, combined with increasing longevity and a growing demand that our sense of sight be used to its fullest throughout our lives, has led to a true revolution in eye care. It is this revolution of technology that has touched nearly all of the eye problems that regularly affect us.

Cataracts, for example, can now be removed during a simple, painless outpatient operation that allows many patients to regain a clarity of vision last experienced at age twenty. Glaucoma, still one of the twentieth century's leading causes of blindness, can now successfully be treated through a combination of drugs and surgery. Even such common problems as nearsightedness, farsightedness, and astigmatism, which for generations could only be "treated" by prescription lenses, can now be corrected permanently through a variety of newly developed surgical procedures.

Like other great scientific advances throughout history, the development of these new ophthalmic techniques has followed closely on the heels of a variety of high-tech inventions. Important modern tools such as the operating microscope, laser, diamond knife, cryolathe, pachymeter, and potential acuity meter have all led to breakthroughs that would have been considered impossible only a decade or two ago.

One result of these advances in technique and technology has been the creation of a variety of totally new treatment options for the many vision problems that have plagued man throughout his history. Never before, in fact, have there been so many ways to correct vision, prevent blindness, and even restore lost sight. The concept of "future vision"—long dreamed about but usually considered beyond reach—has at last leaped out of the pages of science fiction and into the realm of scientific fact.

This book is dedicated to explaining the use of these techniques and the furthering of these technologies. Unfortunately, as with so many modern marvels, many of the exciting surgical options that are available today remain unknown to the millions who might benefit from them, in part because some eye surgeons who could pass them along to their patients remain ignorant of their development or unconvinced of their worth. The purpose of this book is to introduce both curious readers and skeptical physicians to the various new ophthalmic procedures which are currently practiced by a small but growing number of ophthalmologists around the world. This introduction, it is hoped, will partially narrow the huge information gap that now surrounds modern eye care.

ADVANCES CREATE NEW OPTIONS

It is critical that we all fully understand the options that are open to us. Of all our senses—sight, hearing, smell, taste, and touch—it may well be argued that perhaps none is as important to our daily existence as the miracle we call sight. A productive and creative life is possible without it, of course, and a great many blind people prove that fact every day. But ours is a world in which good vision is still a critical means of perceiving our surroundings, as well as a fundamental weapon of survival and a crucial instrument of thought. Those who have it do not want to lose it, and those who have lost it want to regain it.

While good vision has become increasingly important to our society, today's growing population of elderly citizens ironically finds itself regularly facing eyesight problems that appeared only occasionally in generations past. We often hear people saying that never before have they known so many friends undergoing cataract operations, or so many acquaintances receiving treatment for glaucoma. It also seems as if more and more of our neighbors and coworkers have turned to prescription lenses to combat their vision problems, but this is less obvious because many now choose to wear contact lenses.

There is a good reason for these perceptions, and many of them are indeed based upon fact. As the average life expectancy for both men and women has increased from forty-nine years in 1900 to nearly seventy-five years today, the variety and severity of the vision problems we experience has also grown. Cataracts and glaucoma, for example, are most common among those over forty; at the turn of this century, most people died before these ailments had a chance to develop. And while nearsightedness and farsightedness may not be on the same upward curve, the ever-growing importance of accurate vision for driving, reading, and entertainment throughout a greatly increased lifespan has magnified the need for vision correction.

As the bulk of our population approaches middle age and the elderly comprise our fastest-growing age group, a strong desire to look and feel young also has affected our expectation of eyesight. Many of us no longer will accept—without a fight—the increasingly poor vision that for years has been associated with aging. And with the recent improvements that have been made in contact lenses and their widespread use today, many of us no longer will accept a lifetime of wearing eyeglasses.

These factors, along with the general medical and scientific thrust forward in recent years, have resulted in an almost incredible series of advances in eye care. The biggest single boost came in 1947 with the fledgling use of the operating microscope. For the first time, ophthalmologists could gain an accurate and closeup view of their patients' eyes. Like most inventions, however, the operating microscope's full potential was hidden by early equipment limitations and it did not come into widespread use until almost thirty years later. The device has become so advanced and commonplace today that at least one model on the market will now respond totally to voice commands, leaving the surgeon's hands free for other important tasks.

Before the development of the operating microscope, eye surgery was performed either under the naked eye or with the aid of loupes, a pair of odd-looking glasses with attachments over each lens that provided a small degree of magnification. The operating microscope, however, at last provided the surgeon with a clear and well-lit view of his patient's eye, thus allowing for the first time a more minute examination that often uncovered problems that might have otherwise gone unnoticed. This new world of super-magnification also led to the eventual use of thinner and less reactive suture material, sharper and smaller needles, and other smaller, more delicate instruments.

Related developments in ophthalmic surgery have continued at a fast and furious pace during the last two decades and high technology has become very much a part of it all. Today, an eye surgeon's examining room may look more like a NASA ground-control station than a typical physician's office. Computers and other high-tech gadgets fill every corner of the room; bright lights, dim lights, blue lights, and red lights now are as much a part of the examination procedure as was the standard Snellen eyechart in years past. In fact, many ophthalmologists have even replaced this well-known hanging eyechart with a completely computerized version that provides much more accurate information and is impossible for bright youngsters to memorize.

THE ULTIMATE OPHTHALMIC TOOL—THE LASER

Perhaps the most intriguing new tool that has now become standard fare for many ophthalmologists is the laser—the ultimate high-tech device whose letters stand for *Light Amplification by Stimulated Emission of Radiation*. First conceived in 1916 by Albert Einstein but remaining little more than an interesting theory for over forty years, it was not until 1960 that Dr. Theodore H. Maiman of Hughes Research Laboratories used a synthetic ruby crystal to create the first laser light.

By the early 1970s, eye surgeons were using lasers to treat the leading cause of blindness in the United States—diabetic retinopathy. Today, ophthalmologists use a variety of different lasers named for the type of gases (argon and krypton) or other materials (neodymium-YAG) that they contain to also treat detached retinas, glaucoma, and the aftereffects of cataract surgery. Their use has become so critical, in fact, that the American Academy of Ophthalmology has called laser surgery "one of the most important developments in ophthalmology in the past decade," in its 1985 informational brochure called "Laser Surgery of the Eye."

In the ophthalmic lasers most commonly used today, a powerful electric current is passed through a tube containing one or more types of gases; energy is then produced and the laser emits a narrow beam of light that can be focused through a microscope. Different lasers are used to treat different eye disorders, with the choice dependent upon the specific problem to be addressed. Their primary advantages include increased precision and safety, a lowered risk of infection, an absence of pain, and the ability to treat a wide variety of eye problems on an outpatient basis.

One of the greatest impacts registered on ophthalmology by the introduction of these high-tech tools and advanced surgical techniques is the increase in safety and success that is now associated with most of these procedures. This is particularly important, especially when we consider that the very idea of eye surgery is often difficult for many would-be patients to accept. For obvious reasons, surgery on an arm or a leg does not sound as frightening as surgery on an eye—after all, it is hard for the patient to imagine anyone operating succesfully on something as small, complicated, and delicate as an eye. Today's microsurgical tools and techniques, however, have been useful in dispelling these fears by helping to make many eye surgeries as routine as the setting of a broken limb.

TODAY'S SPACE-AGE EXAM

The high-tech aspect of today's ophthalmology begins as soon as the patient enters his physician's office. After a series of routine but important questions about the nature of the visit, the ophthalmologist may examine the patient's visual acuity with the aid of an internally lit, high-density computer screen that flashes various letters of the alphabet at the physician's command. Not only does this allow the physician to measure his patient more accurately than he could with a standard Snellen eyechart, it also allows him to perform the evaluation under a variety of different lighting conditions. (The standard eyechart often proved ineffective in the diagnosis of certain problems because it could be used only in the dark; the newer equipment may be used to simulate real-life situations where several vision ailments, such as cataracts, may be more easily detected.)

One of the most common high-tech ophthalmic tools in use today is the *slit lamp* or *biomicroscope,* which may be used next to provide the physician with a magnified view of the front part of his patient's eye. After the patient has positioned her head against the slit lamp's chin rest and head rest, the ophthalmologist looks through the device's twin eyepieces in order to focus a vertical slit of light onto one eye. He can then thoroughly examine that eye's anterior segment—its cornea, iris, and lens—by altering the focus and angle of the light.

Two other important tools are the *tonometer,* which is attached to the slit lamp, and the hand-held *goniscope.* The probelike tonometer is used to measure the eye's intraocular pressure and thus check for the presence of glaucoma; the mirrored goniscope is used to check the eye's fluid drainage, which when blocked also may signal the onset of glaucoma. Both are safe, efficient, and very effective.

A series of other instruments may be used only when earlier tests indicate the possible presence of certain diseases. The physician may perform a retinal examination to uncover any hint of hypertension or diabetes, for example, by using a hand-held device similar to a flashlight called an *ophthalmoscope.* If it appears as if a cataract is present, however, he will have to use a *binocular indirect ophthalmoscope;* this permits an examination of the retina through all but the densest of cataracts. In those cases, the ophthalmologist may use a *B-Scan ultrasound* to ensure that his patient's vision problem is indeed related to a cataract and not some other problem such as retinal detachment. This test usually will be performed after those described below.

If cataracts do appear to be the culprit, two relatively new tests can help the ophthalmologist to determine the probable success of an eventual operation as well as the power of a *permanent intraocular lens (IOL)* that can be implanted at the time of surgery. The first—a *potential acuity meter,* or *PAM*—is mounted on the slit lamp and used to project a tiny eyechart along a beam of light that is one-quarter the diameter of a pin. This light beam can be sent right through an optical window in the cataract and directly onto the patient's retina, allowing her to read the accompanying eyechart as if no cataract were present. Difficulty in reading the chart will alert the physician to the possible presence of some other vision problem, such as macular degeneration.

The second test is a space-age technique that is used in the preparation of cataract surgery and is called *A-Scan biometry*, which is critical in the eventual calculation of the power of the IOL to be implanted. A-Scan biometry allows the physician to measure the length of his patient's eye by sound waves or ultrasound (the shorter the eye, the stronger the implant). Data derived from this test is fed into a computer, which is then used to accurately calculate the power necessary for the implant.

NEW HOPE FOR CATARACT PATIENTS

If a cataract is found to be causing the patient's vision problem, the new ophthalmology offers more hope for a complete and rapid recovery than one could have expected at any other time in history. A cataract is a clouding of the eye's normally transparent crystalline lens. Years ago, cataracts were not even removed until they had grown very dense or "ripe," which meant that for some time the patient was forced to put up with functional blindness in the afflicted eye. It also was the physician alone who determined when the time was right for surgery. Now this decision belongs entirely to the patient, and the technique and technology are so advanced that the simple procedure can be performed effectively at nearly any stage of a cataract's development.

Today, cataract surgery is a painless procedure that does not usually require general anesthesia or hospitalization. A growing number of ophthalmologists can perform the operation right in their own offices, and their patients can undergo surgery without even visiting a hospital. However, as desirable as these two innovations have been, the greatest single contribution to the advancement of cataract treatment is undoubtedly the development of the intraocular lens.

This tiny plastic implant has been in widespread use only since the early 1970s and serves as a permanent replacement for the eye's natural lens. It is placed in the eye during surgery or at any time thereafter and its precise power is determined by computer; this helps to provide the patient with a vision improvement equal to her maximum potential. Many patients, in fact, say that with an IOL implant they can see as well as they did in their youth.

The high-tech methods now being used for cataract removal are in themselves no less amazing and, together with the growing popularity of IOL implants, they have served to revolutionize this very common operation. While the *intracapsular cataract extraction*—the process by which the entire cataract is removed all in one piece—was the standard form for much of this century, it is no longer the first choice of most surgeons. The procedure most commonly used today is known as *extracapsular cataract extraction,* a process in which the surgeon first opens the front part of the patient's lens capsule and then separately removes her nucleus and cortex (the clear back part of the lens capsule is purposely left behind).

Space-age technology has been directly responsible for the increased use of this procedure, which is more efficient than the intracapsular method, at least in part because it requires a smaller initial incision. Extracapsular extraction actually was conceived and performed as long ago as 1745, but it was not until the recent perfection of the operating microscope that tools caught up with technique and the procedure experienced a dramatic resurgence. Still another recent high-tech development that helped to increase its popularity among certain physicians was the invention of an automated probe that is used first to liquify the cataract's nucleus by ultrasound, and then to remove both the nucleus and the cortex.

Lasers, too, have proved to be a tremendous boon to supporters of the extracapsular method. In addition to the other technological limitations that previously hampered the use of this procedure, eye surgeons were long troubled by the fact that at some point following surgery, some 20 percent of all extracapsular patients would experience a clouding or "wrinkling" in the portion of the lens capsule that had been left behind. In years past, this clouding could be remedied only by reopening the eye in a second intraocular operation.

Today, however, the new *YAG laser* has given ophthalmologists a better and safer way to solve this unfortunate but very common aftereffect of cataract surgery. Several million times brighter than an incandescent light bulb, the YAG delivers a 500,000-watt burst of energy in a trillionth of a second. It can be focused very deeply within tissue and, because it passes easily through clear liquid, it has proven ideal for work within a fluid-filled cavity such as the eyeball. Four to six bursts from the YAG laser—in a minute-and-a-half procedure performed right in the physician's office—has been shown to eliminate the clouding problem without the need for hospitalization or an additional intraocular operation.

Despite the great popularity and success of extracapsular extractions, the third and most modern method of cataract removal—known as *phacoemulsification*—actually shows the greatest promise of all. This exciting procedure, which really is an advanced form of the extracapsular method that relies even more heavily on space-age technology and advanced technique, has been in use only since 1967. But because it requires the smallest incision of all three procedures and therefore promises the shortest recovery time, it rapidly has gained favor among the small number of surgeons who possess the proper skill to perform it.

With the aid of a high-tech device similar to that used by extracapsular surgeons who perform an automated cortex removal, phacoemulsification surgeons open the front of the lens capsule and then break up (or emulsify) the eye's hard nucleus with a titanium needle that vibrates back and forth at the incredible rate of 40,000 times per second. The machine is then adjusted so that it can be used to aspirate this almost liquified nucleus, as well as the much softer cortex.

The biggest advantage to this technically demanding procedure is that it requires an incision of only 3.2 millimeters, which is about one-third the size necessary for other forms of cataract extraction. This tiny incision, in addition to the related need for far fewer sutures, ensures an even shorter recovery time than other cataract procedures, and many patients find that they are able to return to their normal activities within the week.

Most cataracts occur as a natural part of the aging process, and in fact fully two-thirds of the population over age sixty will at some time encounter a vision problem resulting from them. Surgery is the only effective way to treat the problem, but with today's modern methods of extraction some 95 percent of the half million Americans who undergo a cataract removal each year can expect to experience an improvement in vision. No longer must cataract patients suffer in darkness. Those who have endured the gradual, depressing loss of eyesight that comes from this problem will readily agree that space-age cataract surgery can truly bestow a "second sight."

REFRACTIVE ERRORS ALSO CAN BE CORRECTED—NEARSIGHTEDNESS, FARSIGHTEDNESS, AND ASTIGMATISM

While cataracts affect the vision of a substantial portion of our elderly population, the so-called "refractive errors"—nearsightedness, farsightedness, and astigmatism—affect a significant percentage of our entire population. More than 100 million Americans struggle daily with prescription lenses in an attempt to correct at least one of these common maladies, and for hundreds of years such treatment was their only hope. Once again, however, high technology and space-age techniques have combined to open up a variety of exciting new options.

In the past few years, a new ophthalmic subspecialty called *refractive keratoplasty* has blossomed almost entirely as a result of the recent proliferation of microsurgical tools and techniques. Today, many of those who rely unhappily on eyeglasses or contact lenses to see clearly now have an opportunity to undergo one of several new surgical procedures offering the possibility of permanent vision correction without dependence upon such cumbersome external aids. Most importantly, perhaps, the various refractive surgeries now in use consist of procedures that do not require general anesthesia or an overnight hospital stay.

Modern instruments have made it possible for specialized eye surgeons to actually "remodel" the shape of their patients' corneas, thus altering this transparent curved membrane at the front of the eye so that it can focus light properly on the retina at the rear of the eye. This remodeling allows a previously misshapen eye to produce a clear and true image that it can then send to the brain, something that in the past could be achieved only through the use of prescription eyeglasses or contact lenses.

The most widely publicized of these procedures is known as *radial keratotomy*, or *RK*, which is used to correct certain low levels of nearsightedness or *myopia*. In this relatively simple outpatient procedure, which can be performed in less than a half hour, the surgeon uses an extremely sharp and controllable diamond knife to make a series of microsurgical incisions in the area surrounding the optic zone on the patient's cornea. These cuts—whose placement and depth have been predetermined by a computerized ultrasonic pachymeter—change the shape of the nearsighted patient's cornea by causing it to first swell peripherally and then flatten centrally. After the operation, light rays entering the eye will focus properly on the retina, thus providing the patient with unassisted clear vision for possibly the first time in his memory.

Since the procedure's introduction in the United States in 1978, more than 150,000 RKs have been performed with great success. As with most eye surgeries, only one eye is operated on at a time and the patient must wear a single contact lens or a clear eyeglass lens on his uncorrected side until the second operation is performed. Since no stitches are involved, however, the healing process is rapid and most patients can resume normal activities immediately following the procedure.

For more extreme cases of nearsightedness, an even more exciting procedure called *myopic keratomileusis* or *MKM* is now available to many patients. MKM can be described most simply as a way of turning the patient's own misshapen cornea into a living contact lens that accurately corrects his vision impairment.

The key to MKM's success is a pair of high-tech tools—the *microkeratome* and the *cryolathe*—although neither would be effective without the accompanying skill of a qualified eye surgeon. After the operating ophthalmologist has sliced off about 60 to 65 percent of his nearsighted patient's cornea with the microkeratome, he transfers this "corneal disk" onto the cryolathe.

This $70,000 device, featuring digital monitors that give precise cutting and reshaping information accurate to one-thousandth of a millimeter, freezes the corneal tissue and then rotates it while the surgeon carves the patient's prescription directly onto it. The reshaped corneal disk is then sewn back onto the patient's eye.

A similar refractive procedure now being used to correct cases of farsightedness or hyperopia is called *hyperopic keratomileusis* or *HKM*. This technique also involves the removal of the patient's cornea—which once again is shaved down to create a living contact lens—and it also can prove successful for those who have had cataracts removed but for one reason or another are not good candidates for either an intraocular lens implant or a contact lens.

The primary difference between these two similar operations is that in MKM the patient's cornea ultimately will be flattened (like it is in the RK procedure) and in HKM it will be steepened centrally. The degree of each reshaping is accurately determined by a computer, however, and so absolutely no measurements are left to chance.

Many patients also suffer from astigmatism, which is a refractive error caused by an unequally curved cornea. This common imperfection often can be surgically corrected by creating a series of incisions with a diamond knife, much like those used in radial keratotomy. This procedure may be performed in conjunction with an RK, MKM or HKM—which, in themselves, rarely will alter a patient's pre-existing astigmatism.

CURING A DISEASE WITH FEW SYMPTOMS— GLAUCOMA

While most cataracts and refractive errors are obvious vision problems that practically cry out for correction, glaucoma is a more insidious eye disorder predominant among those over age forty. Symptoms of this disease, which is marked by an increase in pressure within the eye that eventually can lead to a total loss of vision, usually are not apparent until a great deal of damage already has taken place. Then, it may be too late.

Two out of every hundred people in the affected age

group are threatened by glaucoma, and the disease unfortunately remains one of the leading causes of blindness in the United States despite the fact that when diagnosed early and treated properly, blindness can almost always be prevented. Preliminary examinations and tests performed by such instruments as the ophthalmoscope, tonometer, and goniscope can help an ophthalmologist to determine the presence of glaucoma before irreparable damage has occurred. Once diagnosed, proper treatment is the key to recovery.

There are several different types of glaucoma and the disease is often subdivided into four basic categories. But while all varieties develop differently, each is marked by the common problem of increased intraocular pressure. This buildup of pressure usually results from some sort of congenital or progressive blockage that prevents a clear, naturally occurring liquid called the *aqueous humor* from exiting the eye at the same rate at which it enters. After diagnosis, it is important that any blockage be cleared and allowed to remain that way. Left untreated, glaucoma can destroy the eye's optic nerve and total blindness may result.

Glaucoma can usually be controlled with eye drops taken two to four times a day or by pills taken in various combinations. These medications will often help to decrease the patient's intraocular pressure either by speeding the flow of the aqueous humor that leaves the eye or by slowing the amount of fluid that initially enters. However, since some patients cannot be treated effectively by these drugs—either because their bodies cannot tolerate them or because the medications do not seem to be working properly—the use of a noninvasive form of ophthalmic laser therapy may be necessary to improve fluid drainage and lower the eye's intraocular pressure.

In certain cases of open-angle glaucoma and angle-closure glaucoma, ophthalmologists have found it helpful to utilize the argon laser to create a tiny opening in the iris of the eye in order to allow fluids to circulate properly. The *argon laser* is a low-powered laser that sends a very high electric charge through argon gas and is quickly absorbed by the oxygen-bearing protein in red blood cells called hemoglobin, as well as by pigmented tissue. Its use has been so successful that laser iridotomy has replaced surgical iridotomy in the treatment of angle closure glaucoma, and *laser trabeculoplasty* has replaced surgical trabeculoplasty in the initial treatment of open angle glaucoma.

HELP FOR LESS COMMON PROBLEMS—RETINAL DETACHMENT, DIABETIC RETINOPATHY, AND MACULAR DEGENERATION

High-tech therapy by means of ophthalmic lasers also has proven very successful in the treatment of several other less common eye diseases. These more serious disorders include *retinal tears, diabetic retinopathy,* and *macular degeneration,* and the possibility for total recovery has increased markedly as new technology and techniques have entered the ophthalmic scene.

Detached retinas usually stem from an initial tear or break in the eye's retina, which is the light-sensitive lining at the rear of the eyeball that receives visual images and then sends them along the optic nerve and onto the brain. If this hole becomes large enough, the retina may peel away from its adjoining layer. When this separation results in a major reduction of the retina's blood supply, blindness will most likely result.

Fifty years ago, a diagnosis of retinal detachment almost always meant that the patient would eventually become blind in the afflicted eye. With the advent of the laser and improved methods of detection, however, some 95 percent of those suffering from initial stages of this problem can now expect full recovery. Today, many retinal detachments can be prevented by using the laser to literally "spot-weld" those tiny rips and tears that are present early in this condition.

When detected soon enough, many of the preliminary rips and tears that could lead to retinal detachment are treated with the argon laser on an outpatient basis. If the retina has not fully separated at the time of diagnosis, the ophthalmologist may be able to utilize this laser for a process called *photocoagulation,* which uses the heat of the laser beam to create an adhesive scar that reattaches the retina to its adjoining layer. If total detachment already has occurred, however, additional surgical procedures might have to be employed.

Diabetic retinopathy is a related problem that also may result in blindness, although once again this unfortunate consequence may be prevented through the proper use of today's high-tech ophthalmic procedures. There are basically two forms of this disease, which is generally caused by a breakdown in the structure, chemistry, or circulation of the retina and is marked by the proliferation of diseased blood vessels. One early form of treatment, called *hypophysectomy,* is still occasionally used and involves the removal of all or part of the patient's pituitary gland. Another once-popular method of care, known as *photocoagulation,* is still preferred by some eye surgeons who utilize the intense light of a xenon arc focused on the patient's retina to destroy the diseased blood vessels.

In the high-tech environment of the 1980s, however, new techniques are continuously developed. Just as many eye surgeons had altered their treatment of diabetic retinopathy to include the argon laser, a newer and more promising variation of this therapy appeared. Involving the so-called *dye laser,* which combines argon and krypton beams focused through a dye onto the retina, this space-age tool shows great potential for treating specific retinal problems with a higher degree of accuracy than other methods currently employed. It also shows promise for a variety of additional uses that have yet to be fully explored.

The treatment of macular degeneration, another problem that is frequently found among the elderly, also has improved substantially thanks to the recent advances in ophthalmic technology and technique. This ailment is often marked by a series of small hemorrhages that begin in the macular area of the retina (which is the tiny central spot responsible for much of what we see), and it can cause one's central or reading vision to severely diminish although it rarely leads to total blindness.

As we age, the macula that is present in each of us will degenerate to some degree as a part of the normal aging process; this may result either in a gradual loss of vision (called *dry macular degeneration*) or a rapid one (known as *wet macular degeneration*). After an evaluation to detect the existence and location of abnormal blood vessels by means of a series of photographic techniques called *fluorescein angiography,* an eye surgeon may choose to employ laser therapy to destroy these abnormal blood vessels before any hemorrhaging or scarring that exists is allowed to progress. Such laser treatment can only be utilized if the condition is detected early and no deterioration of the patient's central retina already has occurred. If caught early enough, however, the ophthalmologist may be able to help alleviate this problem with the use of an argon or krypton laser.

COMPLETE UNDERSTANDING IS CRITICAL

In cases of macular degeneration—as with each and every one of the eye disorders discussed in this book—only a qualified ophthalmologist really can determine what methods of treatment should be utilized and what types of therapy are appropriate. You may think you are suffering from one particular disease and request a specific means of treatment, when in fact you actually may be suffering from some entirely different disorder for which your request is actually inadequate or possibly even dangerous. As in other areas of health care, a complete self-diagnosis without a related examination by a qualified physician may serve little purpose other than to raise your anxiety level over a disease or ailment that possibly exists only in your imagination.

So why is it important to understand the diseases that can strike our eyes and ultimately destroy our vision? Why should we keep abreast of the latest in ophthalmic technology and technique? Why should we as patients try to discover all we can about lasers and cryolathes and intraocular lens implants and refractive surgery?

The answer is simple. Many of the exciting changes in eye surgery, which have occurred during the last few decades at a very rapid pace, have left the public and even some ophthalmologists confused and uninformed about the various new instruments and procedures that might be used to help save your sight. Despite the godlike opinion about doctors that many of us have carried throughout our adult lives, no physician is perfect and few are able to keep abreast of all of the momentous developments that have aided their specialties as high-tech advances continuously appear.

It is important, then, for all of us to be as informed as possible about our own health care and treatment. While no layman can be expected to diagnose a cataract, he should be able to recognize the need for such an operation and determine whether the extraction procedure recommended by his physician is the best and most up-to-date available. While he may not fully understand how an intraocular lens implant works, he still should be able to sharply and intelligently question any physician who unequivocally downplays their use and routinely suggests another method of postoperative vision restoration. And while he may not be certain that his nearsightedness can be improved by one of the new refractive surgical procedures, he should be able to discuss these techniques with his ophthalmologist so that an informed and correct decision about their potential for improvement can be made.

By reading this book and attempting to understand the various new options now available for vision improvement, the reader can discover more about the space-age developments in ophthalmology than he could find in any other single source. In addition to this introduction to these advances in technique and technology, however, it remains crucial that he continuously ask pertinent, informed questions, talk to former patients, and seek second opinions when the first one leaves him uncomfortable.

HIGH-TECH IS HERE TO STAY

In ophthalmology, as in other forms of modern medicine, high-tech is here to stay. Computers, operating microscopes, and other fantastic tools have changed the specialty forever. No longer should eye surgeons be able to make unchallenged decisions, operate on old-fashioned assumptions, and keep patients purposely in the dark. No longer should we as patients be able to claim a blissful medical ignorance, refuse to seek a second opinion, and put off treatment because we believe that nothing can be done to solve our particular problem.

In the following chapters, this book will discuss in much greater detail both the eye and the ailments that can affect it. It will describe specific high-tech procedures that have been developed for specific problems and then help you to decide whether these surgical alternatives are right for you. It will spell out the continuing debate between outpatient surgery versus overnight hospitalization, talk about methods of funding these sight-saving procedures, and specify ways that a qualified eye surgeon can be selected with confidence. Finally, it will glimpse into the future and examine the amazing techniques and technology that are still under development but may one day open up even more exciting vision horizons.

Despite their potential benefits, however, controversy tends to surround many of these high-tech procedures at the time they are introduced into mainstream ophthalmology. A small but vocal group of respected eye surgeons with excellent reputations has voiced disapproval with some of the refractive surgeries, for example, and tried to steer their patients into more conventional modes of treatment. The mass media has picked up on this controversy and many patients who could benefit from these space-age techniques, fearing the bad publicity and heeding the conservative advice, refuse to even consider these important and exciting options.

The actual reason why some eye surgeons continue to reject new techniques remains unclear, but several theories can be advanced. Some physicians, trained before the advent of this space-age technology, may simply fear that they themselves cannot handle the new tools. Others, steeped as they are in established medical protocol, may actually fear the more innovative physicians who generally champion these new techniques. And still a third group may fear anything that is new. (While intraocular lens implants are now widely accepted, for example, they were also highly controversial at the time they were introduced.)

There are, of course, other physicians who initially advise against these techniques simply because they legitimately remain unconvinced of their safety and value. Skeptical surgeons who downplay the high-tech treatments for refractive errors usually do so with the firm conviction that they are offering the best advice possible to their patients. They note that long-term research has not been completed on certain techniques, that initial tests on others have been performed under less-than-ideal conditions outside the United States, and that some surgeons have erroneously led their patients to believe that these new procedures are considered 100 percent safe and effective by the entire medical establishment.

As sincere as these objections may be, however, advocates of the new ophthalmology consider them to be misguided. Some procedures have admittedly been employed for just a few years, but how long should we wait—considering the general absence of serious complications—before we accept them? Other procedures have admittedly been developed outside the United States, but are our country's methods of research and experimentation truly the only acceptable ones on earth? And some less-than-honest surgeons have admittedly implied that these new procedures are completely without fault, but is that not more a problem with the offending ophthalmologist than with the space-age techniques themselves?

Although some of those both inside and outside the medical community will continue to downgrade its potential impact, the concept of "future vision" has most definitely arrived. Modern ophthalmology now offers us more choices for vision improvement, blindness prevention, and sight restoration than at any other time in the long and successful history of medicine. Those who are reading this book have already begun to exercise their most important option. It is now up to all of us to make certain that the technology and techniques it describes go on to fulfill their great promise.

Like most of the technologically literate children who were born into the last quarter of the twentieth century, practically each and every one of the rest of us now also has a chance to benefit from the high-tech world that ours has become. And, just as air travel, telephones, televisions, and space flight have become accepted and commonplace, space-age eye surgery also will achieve its rightful and important place in our lives.

2

The Eye—and Those Who Treat It

Throughout history, few marvels of nature have raised as many questions as the process of sight. How does the face of a friend become visible to us? What part does light play? How are sight messages carried to the brain? What does the brain do with this information? In short, *how do we see?*

The technological and medical advances described in Chapter 1 are certainly amazing, but they cannot compare to the incredible natural wonders of the eye itself. Slightly smaller than a golf ball, this astonishing partially external organ contains an almost unfathomable network of highly specialized cells designed specifically to accept incoming light rays and change them into a form that can be used by the brain. The ultimate outcome of this process—vision—has long fascinated observers but remains at least a partial mystery to this day.

It isn't that nobody has tried to discover how we see. On the contrary, almost since the dawn of civilization the eye and vision have thoroughly captured the attention of biologists and physicians, engineers and philosophers, even artists and poets. Despite countless studies, however, the complicated process of sight is still not fully understood. After centuries of examining this remarkable procedure, we now know what happens to light after it enters the eye and understand how images are transmitted to the brain. But once the brain takes over, the manner in which those images become visible to us is somewhat less clear.

MISCONCEPTIONS AND MYTHS

Perhaps this very lack of understanding, sparking an endless series of theories, accounts for the many misconceptions and myths that have developed around the eye. Many people continue to describe those of questionable character as "shifty-eyed." Some remain convinced that bad spells are cast by the "evil eye." Still others refer to the eyes as "windows of the soul" because of their close association with personality. And "an eye for an eye" has been used to justify revenge since biblical times.

Modern-day misconceptions surrounding eyesight may be less dramatic, but they are equally silly and long-lasting. Who has not heard that you can improve your vision by eating carrots? And who has not been told that reading in dim light, going without prescribed eyeglasses, or sitting too close to a television set will harm your eyes? Reputable eye specialists have spent years trying to debunk these superstitions, noting over and over again that they have no basis in truth. Yet these and other false beliefs continue to be passed from generation to generation.

Why have so many misunderstandings surrounded eyesight over the years? It may be precisely because the nature of vision is so hard to explain. Ancient Greeks were able to master the eye's physical anatomy well enough to perform delicate eye surgery, but they never really understood the complexities of vision and therefore were forced to create a far-fetched explanation for the whole mysterious process. Around 500 B.C., it was believed that vision occurred after a series of invisible rays reached out from the eyes to touch objects. No wonder the "evil eye" belief developed and spread!

It was not until some 2,000 years later that this major

misconception about the mechanics of vision was finally put to rest. In 1625, a German Jesuit named Christopher Scheiner removed the coating from the back of an eye of a freshly killed animal. With the eye's transparent inner wall thus exposed, Scheiner was able to look into it from behind and actually see miniature reproductions of all of the objects that were out in front of the eyeball. His experiment thus showed—positively and for the first time—that invisible rays do not travel from the eye to an object. Scheiner proved instead that light rays travel from an object to the eye, and carry with them the image that is ultimately made visible in the brain.

DIFFERENT EYES FOR DIFFERENT TASKS

Building on the work of Scheiner and other pioneers, scientists now know that sight in its simplest form is merely the ability to distinguish light from darkness. They also have learned that over the centuries, the eyes of different life forms have developed for different tasks. Some basic visual systems, like the one keeping plants and flowers aligned with the sun, do not even require an "eye" in the traditional sense. On the other hand, airborne hawks and eagles possess a pair of highly specialized eyes that can locate prey on the ground at a height of a thousand feet. Then there are those animals who see best at night, best during the day, or equally well at both times. There are creatures who use their vision primarily for defense as well as those who use their vision to hunt. There are animals who can see only what's happening at their sides and even a few who can see what's going on behind them.

As man evolved, his eyes and vision changed to meet new needs. Some 300 million years ago, our human ancestors possessed a visual apparatus that consisted of a spot to detect light and little more. Today, our eyes—which physically developed along the lines of the tree-climbing animals because of an ancient need to face forward and look at a point with both eyes at once—are among the earth's most complex and efficient. We can't see as well as a hawk, and we cannot see well underwater or at night. However, we are capable of rapid movement, instantaneous shifts of focus, separation of colors, adaptation to bright or dim light, and the estimation of distance, size, and direction of movement.

And of all the creatures inhabiting the earth, we may be the only one with a visual system capable of fully organizing and understanding the environment without getting bogged down in sheer mechanics. We don't, for example, constantly see our noses or miss things when we blink, two actions that should logically take place. And we don't see only the thousands of colored dots that make up printed photographs, despite their overwhelming presence. Researchers have determined that these and other phenomena occur because our eyes and brain work together to analyze and process the constant stream of images they receive into meaningful messages. Exactly how this all happens is a little less clear.

CLUES TO A COMPLICATED PROCESS

It is understood today that vision is not a single process and that man's precise eyesight is directly linked to his highly developed brain. The first clue to this theory came in 1877 when a German biologist named Franz Boll was conducting a series of experiments involving a frog's eye. Taking the object of his studies from its resting place within a dark closet, Boll noticed the presence of a reddish substance within the eye that quickly faded after exposure to the room's light. After repeating his actions again and again, Boll realized that a chemical change was taking place within the frog's eye after light had entered.

But the process of scientific discovery is a slow one, and the second crucial part of the theory wasn't developed until nearly a hundred years later. In 1959, David H. Hubel and Torsten N. Weisel of Johns Hopkins University were performing an experiment with cats, in which they first inserted a microscopic electrode into the animal's brain to record the activity of a single nerve cell. Next, flashing a light into the cat's eyes, they detected an immediate electrical response within its brain. Together with Boll's experiment on the frog's eye, this helped establish an essential process in vision called *conversion*—Boll detected the conversion of light into chemical reaction, while

Hubel and Weisel had found the signal that stimulates brain cells to "see."

ANATOMY OF THE EYE

The anatomy of the eye itself is a little easier to describe, as is the manner in which it transfers light to the brain. The point at which our eyesight begins, however, is no less extraordinary than the manner in which it ultimately progresses. Especially when we consider that it all happens inside an almost spherical object that is only about .94 of an inch in diameter. The human eye is truly an example of miniaturization at its finest, with all parts linked by the most intricate of connections and protected by the most clever of materials.

Starting from the very outside, the eye's first line of defense is the *eyelid,* followed by a delicate protective lining called the *conjunctiva.* The eyeball itself is nestled in a bony socket called the *orbit,* which encloses it completely except for a frontal opening through which the eye sees, and several rear openings for blood vessels and nerves. The surface of the orbit is lined with a tough protective membrane, and six muscles that help the eye to move are attached to a ligament at the rear of the cavity. Tears, secreted by *lacrimal glands* found under the bone just above the upper and outer portion of the eye, provide lubrication and cleaning before draining off through small tubes called *lacrimal ducts* found at the eye's inner corner.

The interior of the eye is made up of three distinct tissue layers. The first, which protects delicate internal structures, consists of the *sclera* and the *cornea.* The sclera, or white of the eye, is strong, opaque, and semirigid, and it helps maintain the form of the eyeball. The cornea, a transparent "window" that has no blood vessels but more nerves than most body tissues, is often compared to the exterior lens of a camera. Its job is to begin focusing the light that reaches the eye.

The second layer, or *uveal tract,* exists mainly for circulatory and muscular functions. It consists of the *iris* (the colored part around the pupil that permits light to enter), the *ciliary body* (muscles that contract for near or far focusing), and the *choroid* (which carries blood to various parts of the eye).

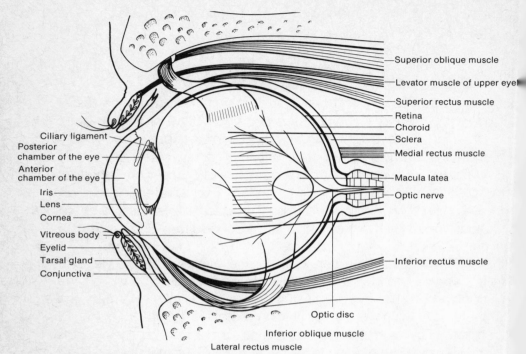

A view of the eye's exterior anatomy illustrates the complicated interconnection of its protective covering, muscles, and other components.

The innermost layer, or *retina*, is a delicate transparent membrane whose role in the vision process is often likened to that of film in a camera. It is attached to the choroid and covers the entire inner surface of the eye, except where light enters in the front. Looking like a pink net and in fact named for the Latin word meaning "net" *(rete)*, the retina serves as an expansion of the optic nerve running to the brain.

There are also three other parts of the eye critical for a thorough understanding of the process of sight. Lying directly behind the cornea at the front of the eye is a fluid called the *aqueous humor,* which is rich in nutrients and helps to preserve the cornea's proper curvature. Next to this fluid on the inside of the eye is the *crystalline lens,* which is slightly smaller than a lima bean and enclosed in a transparent capsule. It serves to further focus the light that has already been partially focused by the cornea. Finally, behind the lens is a jellylike substance called

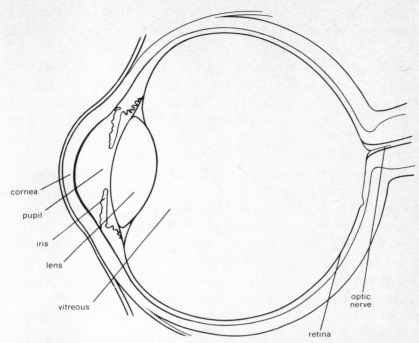

cornea

pupil

iris

lens

vitreous

optic nerve

retina

A side view of the eye's interior anatomy shows the relationship of the many parts necessary for the process of refraction.

the *vitreous humor,* which fills the major portion of the eye's interior and is responsible for maintaining outward pressure and keeping the various layers in proper position and in contact with each other.

NO VISION WITHOUT LIGHT

Despite all this equipment, we still wouldn't have vision without light. What we eventually "see" is actually transmitted by light rays that have reflected off objects within our field of vision. This is why our vision is impaired in heavy fog and obliterated in total darkness. The less light there is, the less well we see.

When these reflected light rays do reach our eye, the first thing they encounter is the cornea. This curved surface—which bulges upward from the surface of the eye like the crystal face of a watch—bends the light sharply inward, and then passes it on through the aqueous humor. From here it is transmitted to the crystalline lens, which bends it further before sending it through the vitreous humor and on to the surface of the retina. Since the retina is not optically clear, the light rays can go no further. Instead, the upside-down and flat image that reaches the retina is transferred to the brain by way of the *optic nerve.*

The manner in which light rays are bent as they pass through the various parts of the eye is a principle known as *refraction,* an English term that comes from the Latin *refractus,* which means to break open or break up. The basic component of vision was not understood until 1621, when Dutch mathematician Willebrord Snell explained why a straight pole that is stuck into water at an angle will no longer appear to be straight. Snell said this was due to the fact that light travels in a straight line through the air but then changes direction when it reaches the water and continues in this new, deflected direction under the water line. He called this process "refraction."

Snell and other researchers soon learned that refraction actually takes place when light passes from one medium to another of different density—like the air and water in the case of the pole. They also discovered that for refraction to take place, light must strike the new medium at an angle, and that the larger the angle, the more the light rays are bent.

Refraction creates effects like mirages and rainbows, and even the impression that a thick-walled glass of liquid looks fuller than it really is. But Snell's observation also had a more immediate impact by leading to an instant improvement in the various optical instruments of his day. Since it was now known that light would bend as it traveled from one medium to another, it followed that a combination of lenses could be used to create the same effect. *Convex lenses* (those with thin edges and thick centers) were used to focus light rays on a single spot; *concave lenses* (thick edges, thin center) were used to spread the rays around. This newfound knowledge would eventually prove useful by helping to accurately correct faulty eyesight through the use of prescription eyeglasses.

After light rays are slowed down and partially focused by the cornea, and have then passed unchanged through the aqueous humor, they encounter the iris/pupil combination. The donut-shaped iris, named for the Greek word for "rainbow," works like the diaphragm of a camera and completely controls the amount of light entering the eye. It is made up of muscles that contract or stretch to increase or decrease the size of the pupil, which sits in an almost direct line with the cornea. The pupil shrinks to sharpen the image for closeup work like reading, and has also been shown to widen slightly in response to pleasurable emotions.

Once the iris/pupil combination admits the proper amount of light, the rays continue on to the lens. This refracting device is highly pliable and can change its shape from flat to convex for various focusing distances. It is also composed of about 2,200 fine layers that cause the traveling light rays to undergo a minute but continuous degree of refraction as they pass through. After this secondary refraction, the light rays then move on through the jellylike vitreous humor, which keeps them on course without further changes.

The traveling, refracted light rays ultimately reach the rear of the eye and the retina, which is a paper-thin membrane lining the inside of the eyeball like a cup or a curved movie screen. Unlike a perfect theater screen, however, the retina has veins and arteries and related areas of greater and lesser sensitivity. Acute vision, for example, takes place only when images fall directly on the center of a slight depression called the *fovea;* another one and a half millimeter-size spot, where optic nerve fibers leave the eye, has no light-responsive cells at all and is actually "blind." But this apparent lack of perfection stops there; researchers have determined that a retina can perform the equivalent of 10 billion calculations per second, compared to a good personal computer, which can perform only about eight million calculations in the same time.

After light has hit the retina, the process of *conversion* takes place and the rays are transferred into partly electrical, partly chemical signals. This process is similar to the one which permits plants to harness light energy. In neither the human nor the plant, however, is this transfer of light to energy direct. In plants, the light must first be transformed into sugars and starches; in humans, it must first be converted into electrochemical reactions. In both forms, this is accomplished by light-sensitive pigments located within the cells.

Within the retina, these light-sensitive photoreceptors are called *rods* and *cones.* Named for their shapes, some 130 million of these photoreceptors line the back of the retina and contain chemicals that are altered when excited by light. Cones, located in the center and capable of sending the clearest signals to the brain, are for daylight vision and to distinguish colors; rods, clustered on the periphery and unable to detect color, are for night vision. Interestingly, the off-center location of these rods is what makes it possible for us to see objects in the dark best by looking at them slightly at an angle rather than straight on.

The rods and cones then transfer light rays into usable strings of nerve impulses, and information about the image's shape, size, color, pattern, and movement is passed along to the brain. What happens next, though, is not perfectly clear. The brain is able to decode and to utilize the information it has received, but how it does this still has not been satisfactorily explained. The mystery of sight—puzzling mankind for centuries—remains at least partially unsolved.

SOME QUESTIONS HAVE BEEN ANSWERED

Over the years, we have answered many of the most nagging questions. We now know how the eye itself functions. We know that while infants are born with the correct visual apparatus, their brains must still learn how to use it. We know of the connections between sight and the sensory system and between sight and the motor system. We also know that a serious brain injury can result in blindness even if the eyes remain in perfect functioning order.

This knowledge has helped us to gain enough of an understanding to pinpoint the causes behind many of the eye ailments and vision impairments that have long plagued mankind. But it didn't happen overnight. There is a great deal of evidence to suggest that the quest to solve man's various eye problems has long been a priority for physicians, scientists, and other researchers. As far back as 3500 B.C., Egypt already had its own medical specialty for the treatment of eye disease, as well as a physician named Ypy who was known as the "Consultant of the Palace to Heal the Sight." Around 1000 B.C., operations for cataracts were being performed in India. And some 2,500 years ago, Hippocrates himself was making references to glaucoma.

EYE CARE TODAY

Today, eye care is far more advanced and complicated, and different aspects are provided by different vision specialists. The primary source for total eye care is usually an ophthalmologist—a medical doctor who has been specially trained to diagnose and treat diseases and defects of the eye. An ophthalmologist has graduated from medical school, completed an internship, and then undergone three to five years of additional training in this field. He is taught to examine eyes in relation to the general health and condition of the body as well as measure changes of vision, determine whether a patient is nearsighted or farsighted, and prescribe corrective lenses for those problems. Additionally, the profession has been divided into several subspecialties.

Some of the same services can also be provided by an *optometrist* (or OD), who is trained to examine and measure eyes for defects of vision, to prescribe corrective lenses, and to grind and fit these lenses. An optometrist is *not* a medical doctor and while he may be able to detect the presence of eye disease, he cannot treat it. For that treatment, the patient must be referred to an ophthalmologist.

The final type of vision specialist available today is an *optician,* who also has not attended medical school nor obtained a medical degree. Opticians do not examine eyes or treat them for disease. They are instead trained to grind and fit the lenses that have been prescribed by an ophthalmologist or optometrist.

This century's medical advances and space-age tools are

two important reasons why we now have so many eye-care options available. But another is our society's constantly increasing longevity; as we live longer, none of our internal systems is immune from age-related breakdown. We naturally develop more problems—including vision problems—that require new and more effective methods of treatment.

The chance for complete recovery from all of these common vision ailments, however, has increased dramatically thanks to the advances of today's ophthalmology. Where only a few decades ago these conditions were often sight-threatening, today they can be safely and effectively treated. And additional tools and techniques are being developed every day.

While eye ailments continue to cause a number of troublesome problems, increasing medical knowledge and constantly improving care offer new hope to the millions who suffer from cataracts, refractive errors, glaucoma, and retinal disorders. A few hundred years ago, these diseases almost always meant a lifetime of less-than-perfect vision. Today, successful high-tech treatments mean that good vision no longer must be sacrificed.

3

New Ways of Removing Cataracts

Cataracts. The mere word—particularly when spoken by an ophthalmologist to one of his patients—is often enough to create a stomach-churning knot of fear and apprehension. Since most of us find the thought of any operation to be somewhat frightening, the very idea of a surgical procedure *within our eye* can be absolutely terrifying. And since many of us also have friends or relatives who have undergone a cataract operation in years past, the still-vivid image of their many inconveniences and aftereffects may be almost too much to bear.

Once again, though, space-age technology and advanced medical techniques have changed the picture dramatically. No longer must patients suffer through long periods of impaired vision as they wait for their cataracts to "ripen" enough for surgery. No longer must they suffer through limited levels of postoperative activity while they wait for their eyes to heal. And no longer must they suffer through inconveniences related to heavy and inadequate cataract spectacles or hard-to-handle contact lenses that once were the only ways to regain even partially acceptable vision.

No, cataract surgery is quite different these days. The inconveniences are fewer, the operation is safer, and the success rate is higher. In fact, it is actually now possible for a sixty-five-year-old patient to undergo a half-hour cataract extraction in an outpatient setting, return to her home that same night, and then play golf within the week.

NEW DEVELOPMENTS LEAD THE WAY

This newfound triumph over cataracts stems from a number of important developments. First, it is now the patient—and not the surgeon—who ultimately determines when the time is right for extraction. This decision, reached in thoughtful consultation with a physician, is based upon the amount of vision loss that is acceptable in terms of the patient's specific profession and lifestyle. A working clock repairman, for example, needs more visual acuity than a retiree who spends his days on the trout stream. These and other patients can assess their actual needs and confidently choose to undergo cataract removal when the time is right for them.

Next, the cataract removal process itself has been greatly improved and updated. It is now a nearly painless operation which usually does not require general anesthesia. In fact, even the operation's once-standard hospital stays are quickly becoming a thing of the past. The federal government and many insurance companies actively discourage inpatient cataract treatment, and a growing number of ophthalmologists now possess the sophisticated equipment that allows them to perform the extraction right in office settings as a half-hour, day-surgical procedure.

Finally, while the introduction of ultrasound and lasers have made an enormous contribution to modern cataract therapy, perhaps the greatest innovation of all has been the perfection of the intraocular lens (IOL). This tiny plastic lens, implanted during surgery or at any time thereafter, permanently replaces the eye's natural lens and permits optimum vision without the use of heavy "bottle glass" cataract spectacles or unmanageable contact lenses. So not only are the inconveniences lessened, but vision actually is improved.

EYE PROBLEMS OF THE ELDERLY

A number of eye ailments are associated with the aging process. One of the most common is *presbyopia,* which occurs in all of us as the eye's crystalline lens loses its flexibility and hardens. After about the the age of forty, our lenses cannot change their shape as easily as they once did and our eyes have increasing difficulty focusing on close objects. This normal condition cannot be reversed but it can be effectively treated with a pair of reading glasses or bifocals that must be replaced about every two years as the lenses continue to harden.

The most troublesome eye problem associated with aging is a *cataract,* which develops when our eye's normally clear crystalline lens—itself consisting of a soft peripheral cortex and a hard central nucleus—becomes so cloudy that light rays cannot be transmitted easily to the retina. This clouding can result from such factors as an injury to the eye, infection, disease, heredity, or birth defects, but the overwhelming majority of cases occur later in life as a natural part of the aging process.

While cataracts themselves are not life-threatening, if severe and left untreated they may lead to total blindness. The only treatment for cataracts is surgery, but the new techniques that are available today have helped to alleviate the problem and approximately 95 percent of those who undergo cataract surgery each year now experience vision improvement.

Recent innovations in cataract treatment are indeed welcome news for the millions of us who develop this common eye ailment, which has been studied for many decades and treated in many ways. Despite the widespread interest and long-time research, however, successful treatment methods were not really developed until recent years. And the cause of the vast majority of cataracts *still* remains unknown.

UNRAVELING THE CATARACT PUZZLE

Despite a cataract's unique and striking appearance—sometimes offering physicians and the patients themselves a clear chance to see the cataract even without the aid of optical instruments—the development of this ailment has long puzzled observers. Researchers still wonder why some cataracts cover just a portion of the eye and then either stop growing or grow so slowly that they only result in relatively minor vision loss, while other cataracts continue progressing until the whole lens becomes opaque and causes a thickening "fog" which can only be penetrated by the very strongest of lights.

Observers have, however, been able to discredit several myths and misconceptions that have long surrounded cataracts and their development. It is now generally acknowledged, for example, that cataracts are not related to cancer and do not result in irreversible blindness. It is known that they do not spread from eye to eye, and are not caused by an overuse of the eyes. Finally, it is also recognized that cataracts are not a film covering the outside of the eye that worsens through continued use of that eye.

Despite some remaining gaps in our knowledge of the problem, physicians have successfully isolated and identified several distinct forms of cataracts and then divided them into two general categories. Those in the first category are called *degenerative cataracts;* these occur when the lens has developed normally but later loses its transparency because of various overt changes. The second group is known as *developmental cataracts;* they occur when normal development of the lens is affected during growth by hereditary, nutritional, or inflammatory changes. Both kinds are treated today in basically the same manner.

The most common form of degenerative cataract is the *senile cataract,* which is the type present in some 90 percent of all cataract patients. This cataract has nothing at all to do with the common definition of senility (a loss of mental facilities), but rather stems directly from the aging process and occurs to some degree in almost all of us over age twenty.

Senile cataracts are usually not diagnosed and treated until they interfere with vision, which may occur from about age forty on. Researchers believe that some people have a genetic predisposition toward these cataracts, and also feel that years of exposure to the ultraviolet radiation of sunlight and the thermal effect of infrared light play a part in their development. The exact cause, however, remains unknown.

Another form of degenerative cataract is the *traumatic cataract,* which can result at any age from an injury to the eye's lens. These cataracts may begin with a hard blow or puncture that penetrates the lens capsule and permits aqueous fluid to enter, as well as an incident that jars the lens enough to cause such damage. Traumatic cataracts have also been found among those in certain occupations (such as glass blowers) where there is constant exposure to intense heat, and among those who have received an electrical shock. In addition, they can stem from chemical burns or even nuclear radiation.

A final common form of degenerative cataract is the *secondary cataract,* which is the occasional by-product of certain diseases or infections such as glaucoma. (Ironically, some of the older drugs used to control glaucoma are also thought to lead to cataracts. These drugs, known as miotic drugs, can sometimes successfully relieve the obstruction causing the pressure build-up and sometimes they can reduce the amount of aqueous secreted into the eye; there are different types for different tasks.) Diabetes is another major source of secondary cataracts, and this type is often called a *sugar cataract.*

The most common form of developmental cataract is the *congenital cataract,* which may be present at birth and appear among children. These can be hereditary or they can be caused by some type of interference in the normal development of the eye's lens during pregnancy. Premature birth, certain medications, or an infection or inflammation (such as German measles) that has affected the mother during early pregnancy may all result in a congenital cataract. One out of every three to four hundred babies is born with congenital cataracts in one or both eyes that may or may not be serious enough to interfere with vision. They are usually discovered by someone

An eye with a cataract will refract light differently than a normal eye because its natural crystalline lens has become cloudy and will not let light rays pass through properly.

who notices that the baby's pupils are white instead of black. Surgery must be performed within the first few months of life in order to ensure that proper visual development occurs and proper mental development follows.

A CENTURIES-OLD PROBLEM

Unlike many vision problems, cataracts have been recognized, if not understood, for several centuries. Their existence was first discovered thousands of years ago in Egypt and then in Greece and Rome. There, early surgeons correctly recognized the problem as a defect of the eye's lens, which for some reason had become opaque and blocked the flow of light. Spotting what they believed to be an obvious problem that could be logically treated (unlike vision ailments such as glaucoma, in which the result was apparent but the cause was not), they were able to concoct a treatment that seemed to resolve the problem. Similar efforts were developed by the primitive people of the Pacific Islands and pre-Columbian Indians of the Andean Highlands.

The word *cataract* itself, however, comes from a complete misconception by these early surgeons that the problem was caused by evil liquids that flowed into the eye. The Greeks called it *hypochyma* and *hypochysis,* meaning "water underneath." The Romans called it *suffusis,* meaning "suffusion or overspreading." In the Middle Ages, Arab physicians translated those terms into one meaning "black water," and their Arabic phrase was eventually translated back into Latin as *cataracta.*

Historically, cataracts were treated most effectively by an

operation called "couching," in which the physician simply pushed the clouded lens out of the patient's line of sight with the aid of a needle that was cautiously inserted through his cornea. The clouded lens thus remained in the eye, but if it was successfully moved it would no longer interfere with the flow of light. Under this treatment, patients frequently recovered some of their vision. Other early treatment methods, which were based primarily on superstition and folk medicine, proved unsuccessful and gradually fell out of use.

SURGICAL TECHNIQUES FINALLY CHANGED

The couching method may have been the most effective means of cataract extraction yet devised, but it was not without its difficulties. These are perhaps outlined best in "De re medicinae," the first complete treatise on the procedure to appear in Western medical literature when it was published by Aurelius Cornelius Celsus around 29 A.D.

Celsus described a patient seated opposite a light and a surgeon who was somewhat elevated. Behind the surgeon stood an assistant, primarily responsible for keeping the patient's head from moving. The only surgical tool involved was a sharp-pointed needle, which was introduced in a straight line from the front of the eye until the physician could no longer feel any resistance. Being careful not to cut any veins, the physician then would move the needle gently up and down in an attempt to force the cataract down below the pupil. If and when he was successful the physician would remove the needle in as straight a line as possible, cover the eye with a wool pad spread with the white of an egg, and then apply a crude anti-inflammatory agent.

While different types of cataract surgery were attempted as far back as 1000 B.C., this couching method proved most successful until a variation was developed in the late sixteenth century. This involved the introduction of a needle through the side of the eye, behind the cornea, which then cut open the capsule that surrounds the lens so the lens could be pushed backward and downward toward the floor of the eye.

Although this method worked relatively well, it occasionally led to a mishap in which the lens was inadvertently pushed forward against the iris—an accident that actually sparked another major improvement. Following a mistake of this type in 1688, a German barber-surgeon named Stephen Blaukaart decided to extract the dislodged lens through an incision he had made in the cornea for just that purpose. This was the first known lens removal, and its phenomenal success rate helped change cataract surgery forever.

After the door for lens removal was opened, other surgeons attempted to refine the technique. A physician named Jacques Daviel reported performing 434 such operations by the time he died in 1762, and of those he claimed to have achieved vision restoration in 380 cases. The procedure was further advanced in the mid–nineteenth century by a physician, Albertus von Graefe, who added the removal of a small section of the iris (now called an *iridectomy* and also performed in glaucoma treatment) to his lens extractions. This saved the iris as a whole from possible damage during the operation, and he reported a 95-percent success rate during a lifetime of some 900 cataract operations.

From those days through the 1960s, very little changed, other than the introduction of cataract glasses or contact lenses to replace the eye's extracted natural lens. All cataract operations essentially involved an incision, removal of the clouded crystalline lens, six or seven stitches to close the wound, and then eight to ten postoperative weeks for the eye to heal. It was all relatively simple, relatively fast, and relatively effective.

Today, however, cataract surgery has been completely modernized and three different variations of the procedure are performed: extracapsular extraction, intracapsular extraction, and phacoemulsification. Despite popular belief, however, cataracts *cannot* be removed by a laser—although the thin, intense beam of light energy from a neodymium-YAG laser is often used *after* about 20 percent of all extracapsular extractions when those patients discover that their lens' capsules have clouded over. Since Professor Danielle Aron-Rosa of Paris' Trousseau Eye Clinic developed the YAG laser, a few bursts can safely and easily slice open a tiny hole in the capsule and lead to immediate visual improvement.

SYMPTOMS OF A CATARACT TO BE AWARE OF

Certain surgeons prefer a specific type of cataract removal, and each variety has its advantages. However, none will prove useful in sight restoration without initially recognizing that a problem exists and then properly diagnosing that problem as a cataract.

No clearly identifiable cause for the development of most cataracts has been uncovered, but over the years a number of common symptoms have been named. Because a cataract does not allow us to see as well as we did in the past, for example, it may leave us feeling that our eyeglasses are constantly dirty. A cataract that is not uniformly opaque or dense may result in double vision. Cataracts may actually cause our eyes to focus improperly and become slightly nearsighted, so we may no longer need prescribed reading glasses. Continuous changes in our eye's troubled lens may lead to consistent and repeated failure of our eyeglass prescriptions. If most of the clouding has developed in the center of the lens, bright lights may cause problems and we may see best on cloudy days. Finally, because the lens' nucleus constantly becomes yellower as a cataract progresses, colors will not seem bright and it may feel as if there is an actual film covering the eye.

If any of these symptoms exist, an immediate visit to the ophthalmologist is advised. There, the patient will be thoroughly tested on a variety of accurate ophthalmic instruments. With prompt attention and proper care, there is no longer a valid reason for anyone to sufffer from vision loss due to cataracts.

Once a patient believes that a cataract is causing his vision problem, it is up to him to decide upon the proper time for its removal. The patient will know he is ready when he can no longer see well enough to perform his regular daily activities, and this decision will usually be based more upon actual symptoms than on examination results. Nonetheless, the patient's physician will balance his vision problems with the cataract's appearance and offer a recommendation for or against surgery. If vision has deteriorated to 20/200 (legal blindness) or worse, however, an operation will most likely be suggested.

It is important for patients to remember that allowing a cataract to progress will *not* affect the outcome of surgery at a later date—except with a *hypermature cataract,* in which the lens rapidly becomes cloudy and fills with fluid. In these cases, all vision may be lost in a few months or even days if surgery is not performed. This is, however, the exception. The majority of cataracts do not inevitably worsen and can remain stable for some time. For this reason, as well as the remote possibility that something could go wrong during surgery, a cataract extraction will usually be performed on only one eye at a time.

TESTING IS PERFORMED FIRST

When a patient visits his ophthalmologist because he feels it may be time to have his cataract removed, a number of tests will first be performed so that the physician can determine whether the problem really stems from a cataract and not some other visual impairment. After checking the patient's eyeglasses to learn if an incorrect prescription may be the actual cause of the problem, the physician then evaluates the patient's intraocular pressure to ensure that glaucoma is not the culprit. The patient's eyes are then dilated to learn whether his vision problem results from a cataract or a retinal disorder; if this still leaves the physician with unanswered questions, an examination with a device called a potential acuity meter, or PAM, is in order.

Macular degeneration—a deterioration of the tiny area of the retina that provides acute vision for close work and reading—is a vision problem that occasionally affects older people at the same time as cataracts. In fact, some 10 percent of those suffering from cataracts dense enough to impair sight also experience serious macular degeneration. Prior to cataract surgery, many patients must therefore be tested for this ailment with the potential acuity meter.

The PAM was developed by two ophthalmologists at Johns Hopkins University, and it permits physicians to determine which problem—cataract or macular degeneration—actually is responsible for their patient's poor vision. Mounted on a slit lamp, the PAM projects a tiny eyechart on a beam of light that travels through the eye and directly on to the retina. If the patient can read this eyechart, a cataract, not a retinal disorder, is the most likely cause of his vision problem. This test, therefore, provides an accurate indication of the patient's potential vision improvement based solely on removal of the cataract. (A low reading on the PAM may signal the existence of macular degeneration and lead to other treatment measures.)

If the patient's problem is determined to come from a cataract, an additional series of diagnostic evaluations are then undertaken in order to calculate the strength of the intraocular lens that will be implanted in the patient's eye following surgery.

A final, important examination is experienced only by some cataract patients. This is an *endothelial cell count,* which is one of the best ways to determine the health of the cornea and to assess its ability to withstand cataract surgery. The exam, necessary only when certain signs are present, is performed by means of an instrument known as an *endothelial cell camera.*

The *endothelium* is a single layer of cells that lines the inside of the cornea. It is designed to prevent fluid from entering the cornea and causing it to swell and lose clarity. All of us are born with a certain amount of these cells; a number of them die naturally as we age, while some 10 to 15 percent of them are lost normally during cataract surgery, whether or not an IOL is implanted. The cornea has only a limited natural ability to replace these dead cells, however, so if the loss prior to surgery has been too severe, special precautions must be taken. Otherwise, even a successful cataract extraction may not provide improved vision.

As cataract surgery has evolved, three distinct methods of administering anesthesia prior to the operation have also been developed. The first and oldest type is a *general anesthesia,* which involves a qualified anesthesiologist's introduction of a sedative by means of intravenous fluids and anesthetic gases.

Applied primarily during inpatient hospital operations, this method is preferred by physicians who for various reasons require that their patients be completely unconscious. Since it also carries with it a mortality rate of one in 10,000, especially among frail, elderly patients, it is often reserved only for those who are particularly upset and anxious over the prospect of eye surgery.

More common during today's outpatient cataract extractions is the use of a *local anesthesia* or a *local-with-standby* combination. The local, administered by an anesthesiologist or an ophthalmologist, involves a sedative first and then two injections—a *lid block* to prevent the eyelids from closing, and a *retrobulbar block* to prevent all pain and movement in the eye. A local-with-standby is similar, except an anesthesiologist is also present to monitor such vital signs as blood pressure, pulse, breathing patterns, and cardiogram, in the event that a problem should occur.

THE INTRACAPSULAR EXTRACTION

Until very recently, the intracapsular extraction method was the most common form of cataract surgery performed throughout the world. Under this procedure, the entire cataract—central nucleus, surrounding cortex, and the capsule that encloses them both—is removed in one piece. This method initially became popular in the early part of the twentieth century, and then grew in use as it was perfected during the last three or four decades.

Patients undergoing this procedure first lie on an operating table where they are covered by a sheet and head drape so that only the afflicted eye is exposed. An operating microscope is then positioned over the eye, allowing the surgeon to see it magnified from four to six times its normal size. After the proper anesthesia has been administered, a V-shaped metal device called a *lid speculum* is inserted between the eyelids to keep the eye open.

To begin the actual procedure, the surgeon places a suture (or stitch) under the muscle at the top of the eye so that this part can be rotated down to the center of the operating field. He next uses a special pair of small scissors, with curved blades that match the eye's curve, to cut back the conjunctiva from the *limbus,* which is an area encircling the eye at the junction of the cornea and sclera. After a groove is made in the sclera with a diamond knife to aid in repositioning the parts after surgery, the ophthalmologist then uses the scissors again to extend the first incision to the left and the right for about 180 degrees.

An assistant then usually steps in to clasp a pair of forceps onto the cornea, which is retracted so that the surgeon will have an unobstructed access to the cataract. Before the 1960s, the next step would involve the surgeon's gentle removal of the cataract by means of another pair of forceps. But in 1961, Polish ophthalmologist Tadeaus Krwawicz invented a device called a *cryoprobe,* whose frozen tip is stuck to the cataract and then pulled from the eye with the cataract still attached. This instrument was popularized in the United States in 1962 by Dr. Charles Kelman, and is now used in nearly all intracapsular extractions.

As the cataract is carefully withdrawn from the eye, the surgeon is cautious not to accidentally remove any vitreous fluid along with it. This side effect is known as *vitreous loss,* and it can increase the future possibility of glaucoma, retinal detachment, and retinal swelling or inflammation. Vitreous loss occurs in less than five percent of all cases, however, and even when it occurs the related problems need not definitely appear.

If the patient so chooses, the surgeon can also implant an *anterior chamber IOL* at this time. These tiny plastic lenses are inserted into the eye's anterior (or front) chamber, the space between the iris and the cornea that is filled with aqueous fluid. Otherwise, cataract spectacles or contact lenses will be fitted at a later date.

The final steps in the painless, forty-minute procedure begin as the ophthalmologist closes his incision by stitching the cornea back to the sclera at the limbus. This closure is made with up to ten stitches of a delicate nylon or silk thread, and is actually one of the most important steps in the entire process because perfect alignment of all parts must be achieved. An antibiotic injection may then be given near the lower eyelid in order to reduce the small possibility of infection, and the patient is fitted with an eyepatch to wear for the next twenty-four hours. Recovery time is around one month.

THE EXTRACAPSULAR EXTRACTION

Although an intracapsular extraction with anterior chamber IOL will usually provide excellent vision improvement, it is no longer the first choice among most cataract surgeons. These ophthalmologists may, for example, recommend an extracapsular extraction with *posterior chamber IOL* as the best possible alternative. Many of today's physicians believe this procedure is far superior to an intracapsular extraction because, in the end, the eye is once again most like it was before the cataract first formed. They also strongly support this method because it usually takes less than an hour to perform and the patient's vision is rapidly restored.

While extracapsular extraction is considered the more modern of these two procedures, it actually is based on the altered method of couching that was first developed nearly two and a half centuries ago by French ophthalmologist Jacques Daviel. Daviel was not the first surgeon to remove cataracts in this manner, but his technique certainly provided the best results. A new and more effective alternative for extracting the eye's clouded lens was thus discovered, although it admittedly was slow to catch on among the world's ophthalmologists. In fact, it took nearly 250 years of advances in technology and technique before it could obtain the status it enjoys today.

In the current version of Daviel's procedure, the patient's pupil is first dilated with about four or five eye drops that are administered approximately ten minutes apart during the hour-and-a-half period preceding surgery. As the iris then dilates, more of the cataract is exposed. This makes it easier for the surgeon to ultimately perform the extracapsular extraction.

In the operating room, everything occurs in much the same manner as it does for an intracapsular extraction, right up to the point of the initial incision. Since in this version of the operation, the surgeon will leave the rear or posterior capsule in the eye and remove the rest of the cataract in parts (front or anterior capsule first, hard nucleus second, and soft cortex last), it is necessary for him to first open the front of the lens capsule. The ophthalmologist creates an initial incision about one-tenth of an inch in length and then continues the procedure by using a small needle to make a dozen or so tiny cuts in the capsule's forward end.

When the ophthalmologist has created an opening in the eye with curved scissors that roughly corresponds to the size of the patient's dilated pupil, he is able to express the nucleus. The resulting opening, about two-thirds the size of an intracapsular incision, is large enough to offer the surgeon an unobstructed access to the cataract's nucleus. He then applies gentle pressure to both the top and bottom of the eye while carefully manipulating the nucleus away from the cortex. This removal is often aided by means of a small instrument known as a *lens loop*.

The cortex must then be removed so that inflammation will not develop, but this important aspect of the extracapsular procedure was neglected by necessity until the invention of the operating microscope permitted closeup views of this portion of the eye. Only then were the following steps made possible.

The cortex is always removed last during an extracapsular extraction and today there are two ways to do this, manually or automatically. In the less complicated manual method, the ophthalmologist uses a hand-held syringe with attached tubing. This device allows the surgeon to transfer fluid into the eye, while literally sucking the cortex out through the tubes. The simultaneous transfer of fluid is critical to the process because it permits the eye to retain its proper shape and volume, even as the cortex is removed.

The automatic alternative, also developed by Dr. Charles Kelman in the 1960s, is a slightly more precise device. In this method, the surgeon utilizes a machine that contains a probe whose tip is entered into the eye between two sutures; by then pressing down on the machine's foot pedal, the ophthalmologist can transfer fluid into the eye at the same rate of speed in which the cortex is sucked out. Successful cortex removal is an essential part of every extracapsular extraction, and the method used, whether automatic or manual, is secondary to the skill with which that method is applied.

In an attempt to minimize the possibility of future retinal detachment and retinal swelling, the posterior or rear of the lens capsule is intentionally left intact inside the eye after this operation. In addition to its preventative purpose, the intact back part of the capsule can also be used to help support a posterior chamber IOL, which is implanted in the space between the iris and the vitreous.

Other Related Procedures

Another procedure that may be performed at this time, as well as during other forms of cataract surgery, is called a *peripheral iridectomy* or *peripheral iridotomy.* This may involve a small cut in the iris or else the removal of a small piece of the iris; both alternatives can be accomplished with a small incision that is often covered by the upper eyelid and therefore not visible to observers. The procedure is necessary because of certain changes to the eye's anatomy that result from cataract surgery. An iridectomy enables the ophthalmologist to create a permanent drainage space for the eye's aqueous fluid and reduces the future possibility of glaucoma.

Recovery from an extracapsular extraction is rapid and vision improvement is excellent. The optic nerve remains deadened from the anesthesia for approximately twelve hours, but patients usually can see very well in about one week after this procedure. Still, they must continue to carefully monitor their activities for a few additional weeks in order for the eye to heal properly.

One final advantage to the extracapsular method is that it will greatly reduce the possibility of vitreous loss and the complications that this can cause. One former disadvantage—a clouding or "wrinkling" of the remaining posterior capsule at some point after surgery—has been alleviated by use of the new neodymium-YAG lasers.

THE FUTURE OF CATARACT SURGERY

While both intracapsular and extracapsular extractions have been used effectively on millions of patients throughout the world, the future of cataract surgery appears to lie with a relatively new process called *phacoemulsification.* This high-tech method of cataract removal, which offers several advantages over previously used techniques, is basically a modified form of extracapsular extraction that differs mainly in the technique used to actually remove the cataract's nucleus.

Developed in 1967 by Dr. Kelman, phacoemulsification is considered superior to earlier procedures primarily because it requires only a very small incision—about one-third the size of a standard cataract incision—thereby providing the quickest recovery time. It has also proven consistently successful in solving the problem of astigmatism that is experienced by many patients after cataract surgery.

After creating a 3.2–millimeter incision—instead of the 10– or 11–millimeter incision necessary in other forms of cataract surgery—the ophthalmologist removes the cataract's nucleus by using the same type of automatic device often used to suck out the cortex in an extracapsular extraction. This time, however, a *titanium needle* serves as the tip of the probe that is attached to the machine.

As in the other extraction techniques, an intraocular lens can be implanted at the same time the cataract is removed. Because IOL technology initially lagged behind the advances in this dramatic new process, pioneering surgeons employing the phacoemulsification technique were at first required to cut a much larger incision than was actually necessary, just so the relatively large IOLs existing at that time could be successfully implanted. This problem has mostly been solved by the recent development and acceptance of newer silicon IOLs, which the surgeon can literally "fold up" and then easily fit through a 3.2–millimeter incision.

The phacoemulsification process, which takes less than a half hour to complete, was initially marred by a relatively high complication rate. Early attempts at the procedure occasionally suffered because some ophthalmologists opted to emulsify the cataract nucleus in the eye's anterior (or forward) chamber, thus threatening the adjacent cornea with possible damage. Today, however, many surgeons choose to "sculpt" the nucleus as far back in the posterior (or rear) chamber as possible, thereby minimizing this potential corneal damage.

In addition to the rapid recovery that follows a cataract extraction by phacoemulsification, this method also presents an ophthalmologist with the perfect opportunity to treat any problem of astigmatism that might already exist. By measuring the patient for astigmatism before the surgical incision is closed, the physician is able to utilize an instrument such as the *Smirmaul operating keratometer* to determine just how tightly the wound's sutures should be adjusted. This not only helps to speed the rehabilitation process, but by tightening or loosening the closure, the surgeon can actually adjust his patient's eye curvature and thereby minimize the astigmatism that is often present in many cataract patients.

Despite its potential, however, not all cataracts can be extracted by this procedure, and only an ophthalmologist can correctly determine if phacoemulsification will ultimately prove most beneficial to his patient. Also, because less than 10 percent of all eye surgeons are currently qualified to perform this technically demanding procedure, only a small percentage of all cataract patients now undergo it. Many practitioners believe it will become the preferred extraction process of the future, however, as more and more ophthalmologists and patients gain familiarity with its benefits and success rate.

REPLACING THE EYE'S LENS

The cataract removal itself is, of course, a critical aspect in the patient's eventual vision improvement, but it still is only one part in the complicated process of extraction and restoration. The patient who undergoes cataract surgery has moved from having a *phakic* eye (meaning with a lens) to an *aphakic* one (without a lens). After this transformation is completed, the patient must be provided with some type of manmade substitute lens in order to once again properly focus his eye. Currently, there are just three basic ways to artificially replace the eye's natural crystalline lens; all have proven effective to some degree, but only one has done so without a variety of drawbacks and inconveniences.

Until about thirty years ago, cataract spectacles were the only available substitute for the eye's natural lens. Heavy and unflattering, these so-called "bottle glasses" looked as if they were at least an inch thick, and they made the patient's eyes appear about twice their normal size. In addition, they also provided a somewhat imperfect restoration of vision: they magnified objects about 25 percent, caused some distortion, and limited the wearer's visual field. But they were still the best alternative to fuzzy vision and most patients were happy just to be able to get their hands on them.

The next big advance in restoring the vision of former cataract patients came with the introduction of hard contact lenses. These lenses offered the chance for improved eyesight without the problems of magnification and distortion, but a whole new round of difficulties soon arose. These included an occasional bout with sensitivity and irritation, as well as a lengthy list of frustrating problems that many elderly first-time contact users unhappily discovered as they simply tried to handle their lenses and install them daily—the actual insertion technique and the manual dexterity it requires (which obviously becomes more difficult with age); and the regime of care and cleaning that must be followed religiously.

Soft contact lenses were introduced in 1971, and they quickly proved more comfortable and easier to wear. But they, too, arrived with their own set of inconveniences. They required even more care than hard lenses, and their flimsier nature made proper handling an even bigger problem. In the late 1970s, the development of special extended-wear lenses that could be left in the eye for as long as four weeks offered a real breakthrough in the problem of handling, but the inconveniences related to lens care only increased because these new models were even more delicate and prone to damage.

IOLs PROVED MOST SUCCESSFUL

The biggest advance of all came around that same time, however, and soon overshadowed the alternative methods. This involved the growing acceptance of permanent intraocular lenses, or IOLs, which are implanted directly in the eye during cataract surgery or at any time thereafter. These revolutionary quarter-inch-long plastic lenses have certainly come in for their share of criticism, but a constantly improving product and a continually improving technique—not to mention a superior vision-correction ability and a virtual absence of problems with handling and care—eventually led to their general acceptance and widespread use.

The first attempt at a permanent implanted lens was made as long ago as 1795 in Italy, but these crude glass versions failed miserably because they sank to the bottom of the eye almost immediately upon insertion. The forerunner to today's IOL was not developed until just after World War II, when a young medical student in London naively asked his teacher when a new lens would be implanted in the eye of a patient undergoing cataract surgery. Dr. Harold Ridley, the teacher, thought about the question for some time before wondering himself why such a procedure had not yet been developed. He then set about the task of creating just such an artificial lens.

The implantation of an intraocular lens, or IOL, changed cataract surgery completely in recent years because it offers patients accurate vision without the problems associated with previous post-operative methods of correction.

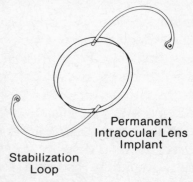

Permanent
Intraocular Lens
Implant

Stabilization
Loop

In 1949, Ridley selected for his new lens a plastic called *polymethylmethacrylate* (*PMMA*). This is the same material which was used to build the canopies of British Spitfire warplanes and Ridley knew that after these canopies were splintered apart by enemy gunfire, this material sometimes entered a pilot's eyes, penetrated his cornea, and became trapped between the cornea and the iris. Ridley—who actually could see these lodged PMMA splinters and immediately realized that they would make a perfect material for his envisioned artificial lens—then developed a protype IOL and implanted it in the eye of a forty-five-year-old patient.

While far from perfect, Ridley's results showed promise and his work was continued by others. During the 1950s, many European eye surgeons tried the British physician's procedure but achieved only limited success. During this decade some two dozen implants were designed and manufactured, and as each one failed, the once-promising process developed an increasingly bad reputation.

The future of implanted lenses eventually took a favorable turn, thanks to the experiments of three men who were actually working independently of each other. England's Peter Choyce, South Africa's Edward Epstein, and the Netherlands' Cornelius Binkhorst each perfected their own lenses that were then used successfully in Europe through 1965, when they were cautiously accepted by some surgeons in the United States. Since that time, results continually improved and implants have become increasingly popular. Today, it is estimated that from 75 to 90 percent of all cataract surgeries conclude with an IOL implant.

Intraocular lenses are tiny, clear plastic lenses (although some newer ones are being made of silicon) that are permanently inserted into the eye just after the cataract has been removed. They replace the natural lens that the surgeon is extracting and help the cornea to once again focus light rays properly onto the retina. This permits the eye to transmit a clear image to the brain without additional external refraction aids, like glasses or contact lenses.

For the extraction and these implants to succeed, it is critically important that the ophthalmologist completely assess his patient's total eye problems long before cataract surgery is even begun. This will help him determine the exact power of the lens that eventually must be implanted as well as uncover any other eye ailments that exist and should be addressed. The wrong lens may leave a patient worse off than ever, and problems like a detached retina may render cataract removal totally ineffective.

IOLs Have Two Parts

The IOL itself is composed of two parts, the *haptics* (curved loops that hold it in place within the eye) and the *optic* (the plastic center that does the focusing work). Implants require no stitches and after installation they remain permanently in place, usually providing the patient with good vision for the rest of his lifetime. IOLs need no maintenance, cannot be felt, and cannot be seen by others.

There are three basic types of IOLs, and each is used in different procedures. The first is an *anterior chamber implant,* which is inserted into the fluid-filled space between the iris and the cornea after intracapsular extraction; the optic is placed in front of the pupil and the haptics are lodged into the angle between the iris and cornea. The second is a *posterior chamber implant,* which is placed between the iris and the vitreous humor after extracapsular extraction; the haptics of these are lodged in the crevice behind the iris or into the lens capsule itself. The third kind is the *iris-supported implant,* which was popular in the late 1970s but has become almost obsolete as the other two were improved; these IOLs were attached directly to the iris so they would not move.

Still more exciting advances are on the horizon for cataract surgery, such as the revolutionary new silicon IOLs that fold up and permit ophthalmologists to properly utilize the process of phacoemulsification. Continuous improvements in operating microscopes, lasers, computers, and other high-tech machinery promise even more advances in the years ahead.

BETTER HEALTH CARE A NECESSITY

The world's population is continually growing older, and as it does, more and more cataracts will be uncovered and more and more surgeries will be performed. As our society's average age and related physical problems increase, the importance of doing all we can to help maintain useful vision among our older citizens also grows in importance. While only about 12 percent of the population is currently over age sixty-five, this age group represents more than 50 percent of all of America's blind. Predictably, a lack of good vision can often leave an elderly person helpless and depressed, and may even trigger an otherwise needless relocation to a nursing facility.

In addition to these problems, a large number of those in the prime cataract age group are often subjected to economic hardship. Many rely on fixed incomes and depend on a health-insurance system that does not even come close to meeting their current medical needs. According to a 1985–86 report prepared by the U.S. Senate Special Committee on Aging and several private groups, the median income for men over sixty-five during one recent year was $9,766, while for women that age it was $5,599. At the same time, the average out-of-pocket expenses for this group's medical care was $1,059 annually. Obviously, this inequity means that a large number of pressing medical ailments will probably go untreated.

Despite the uphill battle, these economic and social problems must not be allowed to interfere with America's health care. As the population continues to edge upward in age, some solutions must be found. In just a few years, after all, the oldest members of the huge baby-boom generation will be nearing an age when many of these medical problems become commonplace. Waiting until that happens will be too late.

The dissemination of complete and accurate health-care information to all potential patients is the first step in ensuring the proper delivery of that care; this must be undertaken jointly by the schools, the medical community, and the media. The continued financial and community support of medical facilities that provide subsidized care for the indigent is another vital key toward this goal. In addition, our Medicare program must be fortified, and out-of-pocket medical expenses for the elderly must be kept realistic. These suggestions will not be easy to implement during an age of budget cutting and government frugality, but without them many of us will be forced to spend our later years without the benefit of necessary care, despite the amazing technology available today.

Eye care is one aspect of health maintenance that should never be neglected, for it is only through a diligent program of timely examination and treatment that many unnecessary vision problems can be found and treated. Cataracts, striking a majority of our society's elderly, are a prime target. Ignored, they can lead to vision loss. Properly diagnosed and treated, they are nothing to fear.

Thanks to the impressive array of space-age technology and techniques now available, the mere development of a cataract should not spark the kind of apprehension and alarm that it once did. The removal of the eye's cloudy natural lens is now a relatively simple and painless procedure that has been perfected over millions of operations.

Fortunately, the existence of a cataract no longer guarantees a lifetime of inadequate vision. And it no longer means inconvenience, either before or after surgery. It is simply one more problem that has been successfully conquered by modern ophthalmic science.

4

The New Refractive Surgery:

Nearsightedness,

Farsightedness, and

Astigmatism

For some seven centuries now, researchers have recognized and understood a number of common vision ailments. But up until recently, the only successful treatment ever developed for a few of those most frequently occurring—namely nearsightedness, farsightedness, and astigmatism—was a pair of specially prescribed corrective lenses. (These three well-known eye problems, present to some degree in most of us, are collectively referred to as *refractive errors.*) Such lenses gradually took their place as the accepted, standard method of vision correction.

Refractive errors are the primary reason why approximately 100 million Americans must rely on eyeglasses or contact lenses in order to see clearly. However, thanks to space-age technology and the work of a few pioneering eye surgeons, we may be the last generation to use these devices.

Since as much as 85 percent of all the information we receive is processed through our eyes, corrective lenses *do* offer a number of obvious and undeniable benefits. Many of us could see a book without them, but not read the words that are

59

printed on its pages. We could see a television set from across the room, but the picture we receive might be fuzzy. And we could see a football field pretty well—even from the cheap seats—but we'd never know which player has the ball.

On the other hand, corrective lenses certainly have their disadvantages. Eyeglasses can be scratched or cracked, and their frames can get broken. They can be lost or stolen, and they are expensive to replace. They can get wet in the rain, fogged up in the heat, and icy in the snow. They tend to slide down our noses at the most inappropriate times and their frames occasionally obscure our peripheral vision. Furthermore, eyeglasses are still unfairly associated with such traits as weakness and bookishness, and many of us have therefore grown to believe that they will affect our appearance and acceptance in an undesirable manner.

Contact lenses, while not carrying the same negative stigma as eyeglasses because of their near-invisibility, also have their drawbacks. They, too, are expensive. They can be very easily ripped and even more easily misplaced. While rain, heat, and snow present few problems, wind often provides a tearful reminder of their existence. Improperly fitted or irregularly checked, they can cause serious infection and inflammation. In certain areas, the dry climate may make it difficult to wear some of the newer varieties with comfort. Then, of course, there are those times (normally while trying to navigate a busy freeway) when for no apparent reason they simply decide to pop out.

NEW OPTIONS NOW AVAILABLE

Still, until the late 1970s, those who suffered from a refractive error knew that such corrective lenses were their only hope. (A fourth related problem—presbyopia, which eventually affects most of us and stems from the aging eye's increasing inability to focus on close objects—also is treated by prescribed reading glasses.) It used to be simple: We either wore corrective lenses, or we did not see clearly. It was either eyeglasses or contact lenses, or life in a blurry world.

No longer is that choice the only choice. Now, because of a series of recently developed ophthalmic techniques and technological advances, there are a number of viable alternatives to traditional vision correction. Virtually anyone suffering from a refractive error today can choose to undergo one of several new surgical procedures designed to permanently correct it and thus eliminate forever their dependence on either eyeglasses or contact lenses.

In order to understand how these new high-tech procedures can be used to correct refractive errors, it is important to first know how these common problems affect vision. It is then much easier to comprehend how an ophthalmologist will be able to surgically help his patient to see well without external aids.

THE REFRACTION PROCESS

To see properly, rays of light must pass through the eye on a clearly defined journey to the brain. As it moves through the eyeball on its way to the optic nerve, the light undergoes a process known as *refraction.* Each part of the eye—as well as its very composition, shape, size, and position—is responsible for a specific portion of this process, and any deviation or imperfection may cause the optic nerve to eventually transmit a scattered signal to the brain. These scattered signals are then detected as the visual errors for which some type of correction may be necessary.

On this journey to the brain, light passes first through the eye's curved, clear, and transparent cornea. The cornea is responsible for slowing down the speed of the light rays by about 25 percent while also bending them sharply inward, much like the path that a coin will appear to take when it is tossed toward a cup lying inside a bucket of liquid. When the tightly clustered light rays finally emerge from the rear of the cornea, they next pass through the aqueous humor. This liquid portion of the eye helps advance the light rays on their journey, but is optically matched to the cornea so as to cause no additional refraction.

The light then passes through the crystalline lens, a highly flexible bean-shaped object that is composed of more than 2,000 fine layers called *lamellae.* As light moves through each of these layers, which lie atop one another, it undergoes an additional series of minute refractions. When the light rays have completed this part of the process, now more sharply focused than ever, they travel through the vitreous humor. Much like the job of the aqueous humor before it, this jellylike substance, with about the same refractive index as the lens, is responsible for keeping the light on its course without bending it further.

Finally, the refracted light rays arrive at the end of the eyeball that is most critical to vision—the retina. This paper-thin, curved membrane is designed specifically to receive the light rays that have been focused by the cornea and the lens, and then transform them into signals that can be transmitted through the optic nerve and on to the brain. As one can easily see, this is a very complicated process that offers many opportunities for something to go wrong along the way. It is something of a miracle, in fact, that it usually works as well as it does.

A normal, or *emmetropic* eyeball is slightly longer from front to back than from side to side or top to bottom. Very few of us can claim such a well-proportioned eyeball, however, just as few of us can claim a perfectly proportioned ear, leg, or hand. Sometimes, the eye's deviation from this so-called norm is so slight that the brain can make a necessary adjustment and internally clear up the signal that it has received. In these cases,

Because light rays do not focus properly when they pass through nearsighted and farsighted eyes, patients who suffer from these "refractive errors" must obtain corrective lenses or undergo refractive surgery in order to see normally.

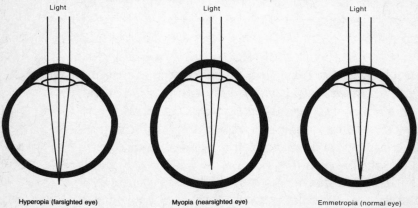

Hyperopia (farsighted eye)   Myopia (nearsighted eye)   Emmetropia (normal eye)

the eye's less-than-perfect shape will result in absolutely no perceptible effect on vision.

At other times, though, the imperfections are simply too great and one of the common refractive errors will result. Major symptoms of these problems include decreased vision, eye discomfort, or eyestrain.

HOW ERRORS ARE CAUSED

Astigmatism

The most common of these errors is *astigmatism*, named for the Greek word meaning "without a point." This condition, often caused by an irregularity or distortion in the cornea, is usually inherited and present at birth. While most of us suffer from astigmatism to some extent, it is often a minor problem. Only about 15 percent of all cases of astigmatism result in blurred vision that is serious enough to require an external correction with prescription lenses.

For proper, nonastigmatic vision, the cornea should be smooth and equally curved in all directions; otherwise, light rays that pass through it will be unequally bent and will not form sharp points on the retina. If the cornea is curved more in one direction than another, the end result may be similar to the effect achieved by a dramatically curved carnival mirror. If the cornea contains a series of tiny flaws, raised areas, or depressions, an imperfect refraction may also result. If either of these common defects are severe enough and left uncorrected, a distorted image will be passed through the eyeball and then picked up by the retina for transmission to the brain.

Nearsightedness

Nearsightedness, or *myopia,* is a related condition that occurs when the eyeball itself is significantly longer than normal and the retina is located too far to the back of the eye. Because this longer eye is more oval than round, the lens, which functions normally and is able to refract light rays correctly, is only capable of properly focusing light from nearby objects on the retina. Refracted light rays from distant objects will incorrectly begin to cross and diverge by the time they reach the retina. Unless this error is somehow corrected, a distorted image will again be sent to the brain.

Nearsightedness is usually an inherited condition that first becomes evident from about ages eight through twelve. The problem increases as the body (including the eye) grows, and then generally stablizes around the age of twenty-one when the patient reaches full physical maturity. A rarer form of adult myopia may develop in patients in their early twenties.

Those suffering from this refractive error usually can see objects clearly only when they are located from about nine inches to two feet in front of them; objects at other distances may appear to be totally out of focus and are sometimes blurred beyond recognition. Because nearsighted people tend to squint to see distant objects, the name *myopia* was drawn from the Greek word for "closed eyes."

Farsightedness

Farsightedness, or *hyperopia,* is caused by just the opposite physical problem. In this condition, the eyeball is abnormally short and the retina is located too far forward. This does not prevent the light rays from distant objects from reaching the retina in sharp focus, but it will cause the refracted light from nearby objects to head for a focal point somewhere behind the retina's actual position. Since light rays cannot pass through the retina, their incomplete focus at the point of impact will provide the scattered message that is sent along the optic nerve and on to the brain.

The effect of farsightedness on vision, however, is not the exact opposite of nearsightedness and is a bit more difficult to explain. Hyperopia usually causes distant objects to be seen clearly while closeup objects are blurred, although farsighted children often can see well at both distances because their natural lenses are strong enough to compensate for the shortness of their eyes. Adults with hyperopia, on the other hand, often cannot see well at either distance without prescribed lenses.

Hyperopia, too, is inherited in most cases, and nearly all young children suffer from this refractive error to some degree. Symptoms in youngsters may include headaches and a lack of interest in reading, but the condition often lessens as the body grows and the eye becomes longer.

AT-HOME VISION TESTS

The major refractive errors offer a clearly identifiable series of symptoms that can be easily detected at home by any careful patient, thus offering the opportunity to undertake necessary corrective measures in a timely manner, either through the use of prescription lenses or dramatic new surgical procedures. By using the charts that are reprinted below, both near and distant vision can be monitored at home. A patient can thereby check for the existence of new refractive errors or for a change in an existing prescription.

Such self-testing techniques, however, should never be seen as a substitute for a complete examination by an ophthalmologist. Only an appropriate medical evaluation can accurately determine the specific nature of any vision complaint.

To test your own near vision, use the chart illustrated here with the help of an assistant. Take the test in a well-lighted room with no glare, wearing your prescription lenses only if they are required for reading. Keep both eyes open and hold the testing chart about fourteen inches from your eyes. First read the sentence on the chart aloud and have your helper write it down, then tell him in which direction the opening of each "C" is fac-

This chart, when used in connection with the directions offered in the text, will help a patient test his own near vision.

C O O Ɔ O   C O O Ɔ O

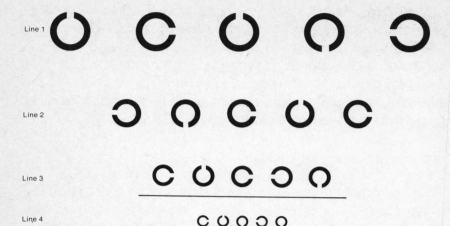

This chart, when used in connection with the directions offered in the text, will help a patient test his own far vision.

ing. If you fail to get the sentence and all the "C"s correct, try the test on another day. If you fail a second time, arrange for a professional eye exam.

To test your own far vision, use the chart illustrated here with the help of an assistant. Take the test in a well-lighted room with no glare, wearing your prescription lenses only if they are required for distance. Attach the testing chart to a bare wall or door at eye level, then mark off a spot ten feet from the chart. Stand facing the chart with your heels on the marked spot and lightly cover your left eye. Keep both eyes open and tell your helper in which direction the opening of each "C" is facing, starting with the largest and working toward the smallest. Next, repeat the process with your right eye lightly covered. If you fail to get all of the "C"s correct on the second smallest row, try the test on another day. If you fail a second time, arrange for an eye exam.

TRADITIONAL CORRECTION FOR REFRACTIVE ERRORS

Historically, all of these refractive errors could be dealt with only by the use of corrective lenses. In fact, until just a few years ago, absolutely no alternative treatment was available. Lenses with a "wave" similiar to that found in a distorted cornea would be prescribed to neutralize astigmatism. Concave lenses, which help bend light rays outward, would be ordered for near-sighted patients. Convex lenses, which bring the light rays together, would be fitted for farsighted patients.

The use of eyeglasses to correct these common problems is so elementary, in fact, that their history can be traced back to a time even before the eye was fully understood. Spectacles were being used in northern Italy and China by the thirteenth century, and Franciscan scholar Roger Bacon wrote in 1278 about using convex crystal or glass to make letters appear larger. Gutenberg's fifteenth-century invention of movable type—and the upsurge in written communication that followed—created a new need for corrective lenses. Surprisingly, however, their use was still frowned upon by many until the eighteenth century.

For hundreds of years little changed in the way these spectacles were designed or used. The next major adaptation occurred in 1780 when Benjamin Franklin created the first pair of bifocals to aid people whose eyes did not focus properly at either near or far distance. From that point until the middle of this century, though, eyeglasses were eyeglasses and their use remained mandatory for those of us who wanted to see correctly despite suffering from one or another of the refractive errors.

The First Modern Alternative

Then, in the late 1940s, millions of people were offered their first widespread taste of freedom from glasses. Hard contact lenses—which actually were conceived in 1827 and had already been available in a somewhat unsatisfactory form for more than three decades—finally appeared in the general marketplace. These tiny plastic lenses were designed to float on the layer of tears (or *lacrimal fluid*) that covers the cornea, to be held in place by surface tension, and to correct the eye's refractive error.

While early models had undergone enough improvement

to make them feasible for popular use by the mid-1950s, many still found these prehistoric versions to be almost unbearably uncomfortable. But the desire for an alternative to spectacles was so strong that as word of these new lenses spread, acceptance followed. Eventually, they took the public by storm.

Excitement over these new "invisible glasses" grew consistently and additional improvements soon appeared to meet the ever increasing demand. The much easier-to-wear soft lenses first hit the market in 1971. Despite their high initial and replacement costs, rigorous care requirements, and occasionally poor vision correction, their overall comfort and convenience soon made them the contact lens of choice.

These soft lenses still had to be inserted in the eye each morning and removed each night, however, and for those of us with dexterity problems, the daily ritual often proved to be an insurmountable barrier. So it was with much fanfare and relief in 1979 that the next horizon—extended-wear lenses, which actually could be worn continuously for up to four weeks—received U.S. Food and Drug Administration approval. These newer variations of the soft lens already had undergone several years of use and experimentation in Europe and Americans took to them avidly. For the first time in history, many of those who suffered from refractive errors found that they could at last live their lives without eyeglasses.

While the contact lens options popularized during the 1970s certainly provided eyeglass wearers of the world with a variety of new alternatives for convenient and accurate vision correction, they certainly did not come without their problems. The most troubling involved the extended-wear lenses, which were so easy to leave inserted that many wearers ignored their physician's advice and "forgot" to remove them at the required times. This occasionally resulted in an infection or inflammation that was highly publicized and tended to obscure the benefits that could be derived from the lenses if they were simply used properly. In addition, these lenses still had to be inserted and removed eventually, and those who were unable to perform such tasks found themselves again left out in the cold.

These realizations troubled a number of potential contact

lens wearers and some began to reject the very idea of using these tiny plastic lenses. Since the general public had already discovered that there were indeed ways to improve vision without traditional spectacles, however, there was no turning back. The widespread demand for even newer and more convenient methods of vision correction continued.

A New Option Appears

Prodded in part by this increasing public demand and in part by the space-age technology that already had been embraced by the ophthalmic community, another development soon surfaced that promised to become even more significant. Ophthalmologists from around the world were starting to praise a series of permanent surgical corrections for many common vision ailments, which appeared to totally eliminate the need for eyeglasses *or* contact lenses. By the beginning of the 1980s, these radical approaches to the treatment of refractive errors were making a cautious appearance around the United States.

One immediate outcome of this ongoing research and experimentation was the creation of an entirely new field of ophthalmic surgery. Called *refractive keratoplasty,* this ophthalmic subspecialty is composed of surgeons who correct certain refractive errors by literally changing the power of the patient's cornea, and thus either eliminate or greatly reduce the need for any external vision aids. In some procedures, they use an extremely sharp diamond knife to cut the cornea and change its shape. In others, they remove a part of the cornea, freeze it, shave a portion to change its curvature, defrost it, and then sew it back into position. In still others, they insert an extra section of tissue into the center of the cornea in order to alter its shape.

A variety of these space-age techniques have since emerged for different ailments, and they have been tagged with such unusual-sounding names as *radial keratotomy, myopic keratomileusis, hyperopic keratomileusis,* and *epikeratophakia.* While these new procedures may still be mysterious to many, their introduction generally has been recognized as the most important step forward in the treatment of refractive errors since Roger Bacon penned his treatise "Optical Science" more than seven hundred years ago.

Despite the exciting potential, however, not everyone who currently wears eyeglasses or contact lenses may be able to benefit from these new techniques. The procedures cannot, for example, be used to help those who suffer from presbyopia. They also cannot be performed on diseased corneas and they cannot be used to improve on a patient's best corrected vision; in other words, most of us with a preoperative eyesight potential of 20/40 still will see no better than 20/40 following surgery. One prominant exception to this category concerns those who were previously suffering from a high degree of myopia but find their visual images magnified—and consequently their vision improved slightly—after undergoing refractive surgery.

CORRECTION THROUGH SURGERY

Virtually anyone else who wants to see clearly without glasses or contacts may prove to be a good candidate. Patients who are nearsighted, farsighted, or astigmatic can undergo a procedure especially designed for them. Those who already have had a cataract removed, but are unable to wear contact lenses and do not desire an intraocular lens implant, can have their cornea reshaped for permanent vision correction. Even a child with congenital cataracts—who has undergone cataract surgery—can be surgically corrected, although because a young person's prescription can change rapidly it is often better to postpone refractive surgery until after they reach their teens.

The first of these exciting surgical alternatives to reach the United States was introduced here in 1977. That initial procedure was designed by Dr. Jose Barraquer of Bogota, Colombia, who had spent more than two decades developing the proper technology and necessary techniques and who remains an important figure in the field to this day. While the American ophthalmological community was initially somewhat skeptical, enthusiasm for Barraquer's technique and related procedures soon started to build.

After several years of cautious experimentation in many parts of this country, as well as additional advances in both procedure and instrumentation, the widespread enthusiasm that is found in many circles today began to appear. Most of the early technical difficulties associated with these surgeries have now been eliminated, and in the proper hands these procedures have proven safe and effective. Still, since surgery is involved, a decision to employ these procedures must be made carefully by the patient in consultation with his physician.

Perhaps the most widely known and practiced of these new procedures is radial keratotomy. This highly publicized operation, which can be performed in less than a half hour, has proven very successful in correcting certain minor levels of nearsightedness as well as any accompanying astigmatism. More than 90 percent of the patients who undergo it can expect to obtain an eventual vision measurement of 20/40 or better, which will permit them to drive a car without additional correction.

An eye surgeon performing radial keratotomy will make spoke-shaped or radial incisions in the patient's cornea so he can flatten it and correct its shape.

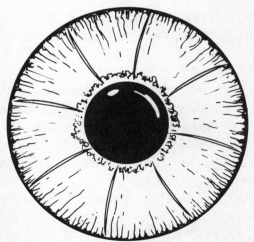

As it is performed today, the surgeon flattens the curve of his patient's cornea with a series of four to eight radial cuts placed in specific locations around the eye's optical axis. This changes the cornea's shape in a way that is designed to redirect the light rays entering the eye so that they can land farther back on the retina and thus provide the patient's brain with a series of clear visual messages.

More commonly known as RK, the procedure initially was conceived by a Japanese ophthalmologist. It was further refined in the U.S.S.R. during the mid-1970s, when a well-known Russian eye surgeon named Dr. Svyatoslav Fyodorov performed over 7,000 such operations. Since its introduction in the United States in 1978, several hundred ophthalmologists have performed more than 150,000 RKs and recorded highly satisfactory results. RKs are usually performed under topical anesthesia only and often on an outpatient basis so that the patient can return home immediately following surgery.

In certain other cases of nearsightedness, a more effective alternative to corrective lenses may be a procedure called myopic keratomileusis, or MKM. This ingenious technique first was introduced in 1977 by Colombia's Dr. Barraquer and to date has been mastered by only a very small number of specially trained keratorefractive eye surgeons. Because of the complexity of this operation, most MKMs are performed in a hospital setting, although the patient still remains awake throughout the procedure and can return home shortly after surgery.

The complicated MKM procedure consists of more than fifty separate steps, and takes about forty-five minutes to complete. Basically, it first involves the surgical removal of a section of the patient's cornea, which is then frozen, reshaped, defrosted, and then stitched back into place. The reshaped or flattened cornea that results, which in just a few weeks will allow most patients to see clearly without corrective lenses for the first time in their lives, is often referred to as a "living contact lens."

A related refractive procedure, now used to successfully treat certain cases of farsightedness in those patients with a healthy cornea, is known as hyperopic keratomileusis, or HKM. Like the MKM technique, HKM initially involves the removal of a part of the patient's cornea. This corneal tissue is then also shaved down and replaced, although this time the surgeon will be reshaping it to compensate for the eye's abnormally short length. His finished product will therefore be bulged or steepened centrally in an attempt to solve the patient's farsightedness by permitting the eye to properly refract incoming light rays.

Some nearsighted patients—especially those who suffer from a condition called *keratoconus,* which is marked by high myopia, high astigmatism, and a thinning of the cornea—may be unable to either wear contact lenses or undergo any of these remarkable refractive procedures. For them, the one possible alternative to corrective lenses is a corneal transplant.

Several other refractive procedures are also being investigated today, although none has yet gained the acceptance and enthusiasm currently accorded to RK, MKM, and HKM. One of these promising techniques, which may eventually prove useful in the correction of certain extreme cases of nearsightedness and farsightedness, is called *epikeratophakia.* In this procedure, the surgeon actually sews an additional level of new tissue directly onto the patient's cornea. This extra thickness, however, has been found to sometimes inhibit the cornea's future nourishment and it may therefore lead to some healing problems. But work on epikeratophakia continues and hope for its future remains high.

Another new technique currently being attempted with some success is the *Ruiz procedure,* which may eventually become more widely used to correct certain cases of astigmatism. Named after Dr. Luis Ruiz, an associate of Dr. Barraquer who is also from Bogota, Colombia, this technique shows more promise than several other similar efforts. It involves using a diamond knife to make a series of incisions in the steepest plane of the patient's unequally curved cornea, thus reducing or eliminating certain cases of pre-existing astigmatism. The Ruiz procedure, as well as a handful of other refractive techniques, is constantly undergoing additional refinements and development.

Radial Keratotomy is the Best Known Surgery

Of all the refractive surgeries being performed today, none has been subject to as much media hype, public attention, and hopeful speculation as radial keratotomy. Televised reports have featured it, newspaper and magazine articles have discussed it, and medical journals have debated it. Physicians, nurses, insurance companies, former patients, and prospective patients have all argued constantly about it. During this time, thousands and thousands of RKs have been performed.

This seemingly unending barrage of publicity has enveloped RK in a blanket of controversy that eventually spilled over to other forms of refractive surgery. While some of the nation's more conservative physicians have taken the position that no such surgical corrections are yet to be trusted, none of them has actually proven that these techniques are either ineffective or inappropriate. On the contrary, the vast majority of those who have already undergone the procedures speak of them with high praise.

To date, radial keratotomy appears to be best suited to those patients whose nearsightedness falls within a certain prescribed but common limit. In other words, if the prospective patient's degree of myopia is either too small or too great, he may not be a good candidate for this particular surgical correction and should possibly investigate one of the alternative procedures. Since the level of nearsightedness that can be improved by RK is subject to interpretation by each individual keratorefractive surgeon, it is best to discuss the procedure and its benefits thoroughly before undergoing it.

Additionally, most refractive surgeons will not perform the operation on any patients who are under eighteen, with many preferring to work only on those already over the age of twenty-one. This decision stems from two important considerations. First, the myopia that is present in very young patients may continue to worsen until they stop growing, which may eventually render the RK's correction ineffective. And two, the younger the patient the more likely it is that the sclera, or white of the eye, will "bounce back" after surgery and thus eliminate any change that the surgeon has made in the cornea. Again, this will serve to negate any surgical correction.

Before it is agreed that RK surgery should be performed at all, it is important for the patient to fully discuss the operation and its potential outcome with his ophthalmologist. This usually includes a detailed discussion on why the patient has chosen to undergo the procedure in the first place and what benefits he may ultimately expect to derive from it. Often, the patient will be able to watch a videotaped version of the actual surgery, and he may wish to contact several previous patients as well as obtain a second surgical opinion. Finally, it will be noted that only one eye will be corrected at a time.

When both the patient and the surgeon are satisfied that the procedure is understood—and that, while no guarantees can be made, it is likely to have a beneficial effect—a detailed preoperative examination will take place. In it, the surgeon first assesses his patient's visual requirement by measuring the eye's corneal thickness on a tabletop instrument called an *ultrasonic pachymeter.* A computer program is then used to determine how many incisions the patient will need for correction, and where these cuts should eventually be placed in his optical zone.

The RK Procedure

The RK operation itself is a relatively simple day-surgical procedure that can be performed on an outpatient basis in either a hospital or approved outpatient clinic. Topical anesthesia (in the form of eye drops) is the anesthesia of choice, unless the patient is particularly anxious and desires an intravenous medication to make him feel more relaxed. General anesthesia also can be used, but the patient will then have to remain in the hospital for a slightly longer period.

Once the patient's eye is anesthetized, he will be wheeled into an operating room and covered with a surgical drape that exposes only the eye to be corrected. His surgeon will be seated at an operating microscope that is positioned above the patient's head, and at least one assistant will be nearby.

Unless a general anesthesia has been requested, the patient will be awake during the entire operation.

The painless procedure itself consists of a series of from four to eight microsurgical incisions around the optic zone that are usually made with a diamond knife. The incisions, whose dimensions have already been determined by a computer in the preoperative examination, are placed in a radial pattern on the surface of the cornea at an average depth of about 90 percent of the cornea's thickness. Although awake, the patient will not be able to either see or feel them.

The purpose of the incisions is to cause the cornea to swell peripherally and then flatten centrally. This change in the patient's previously misshapen cornea will allow the incoming light rays to land back on the retina for clear vision, instead of landing in the middle of the eye and resulting in blurry vision. In effect, the surgeon will be reforming the patient's eye so that it will refract light properly and send more accurate visual images to his brain.

The entire RK operation can take from fifteen to thirty minutes, after which the patient's eye is patched. As long as a general anesthesia has not been used, he soon can return home. Since local anesthesia will deaden the eye's optic nerve for as long as eighteen hours, the patient will feel nothing and in most cases will experience little more than mild discomfort following the surgery. After the anesthesia wears off, there is usually sufficient healing to prevent any additional pain. Since no stitches have been used, the incisions will heal properly on their own.

When the patch is removed on the following day, the patient will see and see well, although there may be a slight blurring of vision due to some initial instability. Other possible side effects include night-time glare, altered depth perception, and the sensation that a foreign body is present in the eye. As the cornea heals and flattens, however, it settles into its correct new curvature and vision is usually stabilized. The surgeon will then measure the eye on several different occasions, and an often steady improvement in vision will be noted.

Because of their particular vision problems, some patients may need to undergo the procedure on only one eye. For the majority of others who are awaiting a second RK, it will be necessary to wear either one contact lens in the uncorrected eye, or else a pair of glasses that has been fitted with a clear lens on the side that was corrected. Eventually, many RK patients will be able to function perfectly well with no corrective lenses at all, although some may later find a pair of reading glasses to be helpful.

Surgery for More Serious Myopia

While radial keratotomy is a relatively simple refractive procedure designed to correct most minor cases of nearsightedness, myopic keratomileusis is a much more complicated technique intended primarily for only the most serious of cases; the kind of people who often need glasses just to find their glasses. A candidate for MKM, for example, may suffer from uncorrected vision as poor as 20/4,000; by way of comparison, a person whose vision is worse than 20/400 cannot read the big "E" at the top of the Snellen eyechart. Nearly 1,000 patients have already undergone MKM, and it is being widely recognized as one of the most ingenious procedures available in eye surgery today.

An ideal candidate for an MKM is the person who suffers from a severe degree of myopia but still possesses a healthy cornea. This potential patient must also be unhappy with both eyeglasses and contact lenses for one of numerous personal or professional reasons. A myopic restaurant chef who is not able to wear contacts comfortably, for example, may be tired of having her glasses steam up in the kitchen. And a nearsighted construction worker may be uneasy with thick glasses, but unable to wear contacts because of the dust that is always present at his job. These are the type of people who may consider an MKM to be beneficial.

As with the RK procedure, most refractive surgeons who practice this technique have set a minimum age limit for their potential MKM patients. Although the procedure can, physically, be performed on an eye of any age, MKM surgeons usually will not consider a patient who is under eighteen unless there is an absolute necessity that the operation be undertaken. And even then other options will probably be explored first.

After attending a counseling session similar to the one conducted with prospective RK patients, the future MKM patient should feel completely at ease with both the surgeon and the technique. A surgeon with no experience in this difficult procedure, for example, may possibly be unable to perform the delicate maneuvers that are required. Likewise, a surgeon who appears clumsy during the examination process will probably not become smooth and coordinated in the operating room.

Once again, the operation itself usually will be performed under local anesthesia. While this prevents the possibility of feeling any pain, the patient will nonetheless remain awake during the entire ninety-minute procedure and be totally conscious of what is happening. Under special circumstances, intravenous medication or even a general anesthesia may again be used.

The MKM Procedure

As the actual surgery is about to begin, an assistant preprograms the computer with information about the patient's eye that has already been obtained. Then the manual portion of the operation gets underway. The surgeon begins by slicing off about 60 to 65 percent of the central portion of the cornea with an instrument known as a *microkeratome*. Although the percentages make it sound as if the surgeon will have a great deal of tissue with which to work, the piece of cornea that has been removed actually is only about the size and thickness of a contact lens.

Operating without rubber gloves in order to avoid getting powdery film on the *corneal interface*—the sticky surface that is exposed after the cornea is cut—the sliced piece of cornea is next transferred onto the cryolathe, which freezes it with a blast of carbon dioxide. This step transforms the human tissue into a rigid disk, so that it can be more easily cut and shaped while it is rotated on the cryolathe. The surgeon then carves the patient's prescription precisely into this piece of cornea, which when completed will serve as a hollowed-out, concave-surface lens that has been accurately reshaped to eliminate the nearsightedness that existed previously.

After the piece of removed corneal tissue has been properly hollowed and reshaped to correct the patient's refractive error, it is defrosted and sutured back into place. A pressure patch is then placed over the eye, which will be worn for two-to three-and-a-half days. Two weeks later, all sutures will be removed. As with most of those who undergo RK, the patient's vision is expected to improve almost daily.

As unbelievable as it may sound, every one of the adjustments that were made during the carving of the tissue has been determined by computer. The surgeon must first feed the computer with the necessary information on the patient's preoperative visual acuity, the desired postoperative correction (which will be zero), and the preoperative corneal curvature. And then, of course, he must be properly skilled in order to actually perform the maneuvers that the computer has determined to be necessary. MKM is truly an example of space-age eye surgery at its finest.

Hyperopic keratomileusis, or HKM, is a very similar procedure that is often used to correct certain cases of farsightedness. During this operation, though, the patient's cornea is carved in a slightly different manner that causes it to bulge out centrally after it is replaced. Both MKM and HKM are used to compensate for the uncorrected eye's own inability to properly refract light rays. The small number of surgeons who currently perform them insist that they work better, and present fewer complications, than any other surgical alternative that could be applied to these patients.

CHOICE OF SURGEON IS CRITICAL

The important thing to remember with any of these procedures, however, is that the choice of a knowledgable and competent surgeon is critical to their eventual success. There are some physicians who tout these high-tech refractive techniques as a cureall for everyone's eye problems, and this is just not the case. There also are some physicians who perform these procedures on suitable patients, but actually handle the surgery improperly. Either way these actions reflect on the entire field of refractive surgery, which can then unfairly develop a bad reputation.

But the amount of positive reactions connected to these procedures generally continues to outweigh the few negative comments that have been voiced. New high-tech devices that help ensure their success are entering the ophthalmic marketplace all the time. In addition, word continues to spread about the potential of these new corrective techniques, which causes more and more of those who suffer from refractive errors to consider undergoing them.

So why do headlines occasionally pop up that offer a skeptical view of the procedures? Why do many highly respected ophthalmologists insist that at best their value has yet to be proven, and at worst they already have been proven ineffective? Why has a widening gap developed between those who support these revolutionary corrective procedures and those who do not?

There are several theories that may offer a reason for this reluctance and rejection. One states that many health-care professionals are often afraid of anything that is new and refractive surgery is certainly new. In addition, a number of ophthalmologists who learned their skills in the days before the computer age are naturally hesitant to utilize the imposing high-tech tools that are critical to this field. A physician who cannot bear to sit down at a personal computer to type a scientific paper, after all, will certainly be opposed to using an even more intricate device to help him operate on a patient's eye.

Then there is the possibility that refractive surgery's high visibility and rapid public acceptance has actually worked against it. Publicity and attention, some physicians may feel, are the mark of Madison Avenue and have no place in medicine. If these procedures are really worthwhile, these critics seem to be saying, they will receive proper attention in the proper manner at the proper time. While this argument is not valid, it may really be behind a great deal of the criticism that is directed toward refractive surgery.

Additionally, some ophthalmologists—who perhaps see their own retirements not too far off and may therefore be content with supporting medicine's status quo—are apparently afraid to rock the medical world's boat. They perhaps feel that many of the eye surgeons who were first to perform these re-fractive procedures are the very ones who often are first in other areas, too. They see these younger professionals aggressively advertising their skills, marketing their practices, and appearing on television and radio to tout the new high-tech procedures. In the minds of the old guard, this just will not do.

Finally, there is the argument that such techniques are in-herently improper because they involve the performance of surgery on an otherwise healthy eye. This may be the oldest ar-gument against such procedures, but it also may be the least rational and persuasive. What is healthy about an eye that can-not see a bird in a tree? What is healthy about a lifetime of in-security often begun with the verbal insults that a youngster with thick glasses often receives from his peers? And what is healthy about a young adult with low self-esteem who hates his eye-glasses so much that he decides to live his life without them, preferring a world of blurry vision to a world of sharpness and definition?

THE DEBATE CONTINUES

Still, some legitimate concerns have been raised. A few critics complain that too many patients decide to undergo these procedures strictly for cosmetic reasons. Others cite the chance that an eye will be accidentally undercorrrected or overcorrected, thus leaving the patient in no better visual shape than before the surgery was attempted. Yet another group notes that the cornea is extremely slow to heal, and that vision fluctuations have been detected in some refractive surgery pa-tients several years after their operation.

Some of the questions related to the effectiveness and safety of radial keratotomy were addressed in an official 1985 position paper issued by the American Academy of Ophthal-mology. (The organization offered no comparable opinion on the more complex MKM and HKM techniques.) Noting that research on RKs had not yet been completed and no definitive statement could therefore be made, the Academy said it was basing its opinion entirely on information that was available.

The one-page Academy paper concludes by calling RK

"an investigational procedure for the modification of myopia which should be conducted in accordance with adequate review mechanisms and preceded by appropriate informed consent which recognizes the special nature and presently uncertain ramifications of the procedure." Nevertheless, the paper notes "that most individuals who have undergone radial keratotomy are pleased with the initial results."

Groups such as the Texas-based Kerato-Refractive Society continue to publicize the positive side of these procedures, and eye surgeons across the nation continue to suggest them to their patients. Advocates claim that, in the proper surgical hands, these techniques are effective and safe. They point to thousands of patients who have undergone the procedures since the late 1970s, and the vast number who would recommend them to others without hesitation. And they hope critics both inside and outside the medical profession will soon accept the fact that these procedures can be beneficial to many patients.

One day, perhaps, all of the medical community will throw its support behind these surgical techniques. Until that time, those who suffer from refractive errors have a couple of distinctly different choices. They can continue to wear eyeglasses or contact lenses, or they can investigate the new high-tech refractive procedures, which will prove beneficial to most, unappealing to some, and inaccessible to a few.

Despite some opposition, these procedures appear to be here to stay, and that is good news for those who suffer from such problems as nearsightedness, farsightedness, and astigmatism. Intraocular lens implants, now considered a standard procedure that safely and routinely follows most cataract operations, are among the numerous high-tech ophthalmic innovations that were also scorned upon their introduction. Even outside the medical field, a countless number of daring scientific advances were denounced before they were finally accepted and eventually became the norm.

The future of vision correction undoubtedly lies with these high-tech refractive procedures.

5

The Pressures of Glaucoma

Of all the eye diseases discussed in this book, glaucoma stands alone. Like some of the other disorders it strikes late in life and may, if untreated, result in total and irreversible blindness. Most common eye ailments lead to an almost immediate vision problem that soon becomes apparent to the observant patient. Glaucoma, however, is not like that at all.

Unlike cataracts, which worsen over time but noticeably impair a patient's vision only gradually as they progress, glaucoma is an insidious disease that literally sneaks up on its victims. Unlike refractive errors, it does not lead to fuzzy vision that can be detected with an eye chart. Unlike certain infections and inflammations, there is rarely any pain. In fact, without a thorough and periodic eye examination specifically designed to detect it, glaucoma will offer few obvious clues to its existence until its damage has been done. Then it is often too late for effective treatment.

Glaucoma is mainly a disease of the middle-aged; it is rarely found among those in their teens or those over seventy. It is fairly common among adults in its primary target group, though, and it affects the vision of about two out of every hundred people over age forty. Black patients, those with a family history of glaucoma, and those suffering from a variety of general health problems such as diabetes, hardening of the arteries, or anemia are particularly at risk. Men and women are equally vulnerable to its onset, and it usually affects both eyes of its victims. Oddly enough, it is found more among farsighted individuals than among those who suffer from nearsightedness.

When glaucoma is diagnosed early and treated properly, the loss of vision that eventually stems from its long-term presence can almost always be prevented. Since its symptoms generally are subtle and hard to detect, however, a correct diagnosis and adequate treatment, critical to stopping its destructive properties, may not be initiated early enough without careful and consistent monitoring. Despite the variety of successful methods of treatment that have been developed over the years, therefore, glaucoma continues to remain one of the leading causes of blindness in the United States.

Glaucoma has been recognized as a serious eye disease for several thousand years, and even Hippocrates, the great Greek physician and acknowledged father of medicine, referred to the disorder some 2,500 years ago. Since the earlier eye surgeons lacked the precise tools and techniques that are available today, it took a great many years before the basic cause of glaucoma was actually uncovered. Many more years then passed before effective methods of treatment were developed.

Today, our knowledge of glaucoma is extensive. Thanks to a variety of microsurgical instruments and high-tech examination procedures, we now know that the disease we call glaucoma actually is a complex of several related disorders of the eye. Despite their differences, each is characterized by an increase in *intraocular pressure,* or *IOP,* which is the force exerted outward by one of two liquids occurring naturally within the eye. If left untreated, this increased pressure can in time prove sufficient to produce significant visual impairment, including but not limited to total blindness.

THE CAUSE OF GLAUCOMA

   Basically, the onset of glaucoma is related to the inability of a transparent liquid constantly circulating within our eyes to drain off properly. This fluid, called aqueous humor, is mostly water. It fills our eye's anterior chamber, the space between the back of the cornea and the front of the iris, and supplies it with various nutrients (including Vitamin C), removes waste products, and assists the cornea in maintaining its proper curvature and shape.

   Aqueous humor is produced by a group of glands called

Aqueous humor normally flows through the eye on a regular basis—unless glaucoma is present and the fluid becomes trapped, thus raising the patient's intraocular pressure.

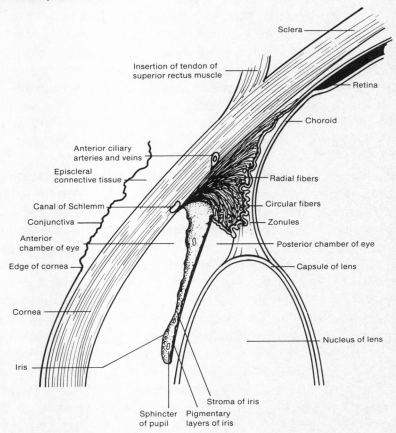

Sclera

Insertion of tendon of
superior rectus muscle

Retina

Choroid

Anterior ciliary
arteries and veins

Episcleral
connective tissue

Radial fibers

Canal of Schlemm

Circular fibers

Conjunctiva

Zonules

Anterior
chamber of eye

Posterior chamber of eye

Edge of cornea

Capsule of lens

Cornea

Nucleus of lens

Iris

Stroma of iris

Sphincter   Pigmentary
of pupil   layers of iris

the *ciliary body* that are found in the part of the eye that adjoins the iris. Normally, this fluid flows continuously into the inner eye after being filtered through several layers of porous fibers named *trabecula;* it then passes continuously out of the eye through a circular channel known as the *Canal of Schlemm.* In the eyes of most of us, this flowing liquid will maintain a constant pressure within the forward chamber that neither increases nor decreases over the passage of time. Sometimes, though, the eye's drainage system becomes stopped up or blocked. When this occurs, the aqueous humor exit can be impaired and pressure inside the eye could increase.

Despite our current high level of knowledge about glaucoma, some aspects of the disease still remain a mystery. We do not know, for example, exactly why several common varieties of the disorder tend to occur in some patients and not in others. The reason for this appears to be the development of some type of obstruction that interferes with the exit of aqueous humor from the eye, rather than any change in the nature of the fluid or an increase in its production. Why this obstruction initially develops, however, is still unclear.

HOW VISION IMPAIRMENT RESULTS

Because of the revolutionary techniques and technology that have allowed us to thoroughly study the eye in recent years, however, we now know how untreated glaucoma can result in vision impairment and blindness. All of the images that are perceived by our eyes as rays of light land eventually on the retina, where they are translated into a series of signals that can be sent along the eye's optic nerve for reception and decoding by the brain. The optic nerve often is likened to a kind of electronic cable that contains millions of tiny nerve fibers or "wires" for transmitting these translated messages, which the retina already has broken down into separate signals for our peripheral vision and our central vision.

If glaucoma is present and the aqueous humor is entering the eye at a faster rate than it can leave, pressure within the eye naturally will increase. This pressure may deform the optic nerve slowly and steadily, while gradually altering the shape of the *optic nerve head*—the point where the optic nerve adjoins the retina, also often called the *optic disc*—until it starts to resemble a deepening cup. While the optic nerve head is suffering this external damage, the "wires" that are inside of the optic nerve itself are continuously atrophying and dying.

As the disease progresses and this cupping becomes more extreme, blind spots will begin to develop in certain areas of the patient's vision. Since the "wires" that handle the signals for our peripheral or side vision are usually the first ones to suffer damage from glaucoma, few of us even notice that our field of vision is gradually diminishing—until, that is, the optic nerve has suffered considerable destruction and our central vision also has begun to worsen. Once the entire optic nerve has been destroyed, however, irreversible blindness almost certainly will result.

Despite the various high-tech treatments for battling glaucoma that have been developed and introduced during the past few decades, no physician as yet has the ability to reverse any damage that already has been sustained by the optic nerve at the point of diagnosis. Therefore, the key to controlling this destructive eye disorder clearly involves early detection. Glaucoma remains responsible for approximately one out of every seven cases of blindness, but this statistic can be changed if those in the primary target group would simply undergo periodic and complete eye examinations.

TESTING FOR GLAUCOMA

Many physicians can offer tests for glaucoma as a part of their regular physical exams, but only an ophthalmologist is specifically equipped and trained to perform an examination for glaucoma and then treat the disease if evidence of its presence is uncovered. Since patients with the most common form of glaucoma rarely suffer from any symptoms other than headaches, these periodic tests must be performed even though no apparent reason for them exists.

One important test in the search for glaucoma involves an

ophthalmoscope, which actually was invented back in 1851 by German scientist Hermann von Helmholtz. This instrument allows the physician to focus a beam of light into his patient's eye and then magnify its reflection. By using an ophthalmoscope the ophthalmologist can examine the interior of his patient's eye in intricate detail and even study the parts that are located far to the back, such as the retina and the optic nerve. This may reveal early signs of cupping and indicate whether glaucoma exists, even though no other symptoms have been noticed.

A second important test for glaucoma is called *goniscopy,* which is a slightly more difficult procedure often requiring the use of a pair of specially made contact lenses, a hand-held illuminator, and a hand-held binocular microscope. With the patient reclining on his back and the special contact lenses placed over his eyes, the physician is then able to thoroughly examine the eyes' anterior or forward chambers. This permits him to see if the base of the patient's iris already blocks or is likely to block the exit of aqueous humor through the Canal of Schlemm. Other systems of performing goniscopy—including the use of mirrored contact lenses and the slit-lamp microscope, employed while the patient is seated—also can produce the desired information.

Perhaps no glaucoma examination, however, is as revealing as the one that utilizes a *tonometer.* This deceptively simple instrument, originally developed in Norway in 1905 by Hjalmar Schiotz, allows the ophthalmologist to accurately measure the pressure within his patient's eyes. If the pressure is above a certain predetermined level—again, even if no additional overt symptoms have been experienced—it becomes apparent to both physician and patient that glaucoma is most likely present.

The original tonometer, called the *Schiotz tonometer* in honor of its inventor, actually is a simple "low-tech" device that still is the most widely used tonometer in the world. With the patient on his back and gazing upward, the physician places a drop of topical anesthetic in the eye to be examined; he then manually places the hand-size Schiotz tonometer directly upon the patient's cornea. The extent to which a weighted plunger on the tonometer is able to indent the cornea is measured on a scale by a simple lever-arm indicator, and the physician quickly can assess the pressure that is being exerted from the inside of the patient's eye. The Schiotz tonometer is convenient and portable, but it is subject to occasional error. This is the chief reason why a newer, high-tech version now is gaining favor among many ophthalmologists.

Called the *Goldmann applanation tonometer,* this new space-age tool usually provides more accurate results than its predecessor. It is so precise, in fact, that it is often used for a backup test by physicians who for one reason or another may question the results of a Schiotz-tonometer examination.

The Goldmann applanation tonometer is a complex piece of modern machinery that is mounted on a slit lamp. For this examination the patient is seated in front of the slit lamp and given a drop of a topical anesthetic followed by a drop of an orange dye called *fluorescein,* which is an ocular tracer that will dissolve into tears and enable the tonometer to pick up images of the patient's eyes as fluorescent yellow-green arcs.

The patient is then instructed to rest his forehead firmly against a bar on the slip lamp and to remain as motionless as possible in that position.

After placing a blue filter in front of the tonometer's light beam, the physician then aligns the device with the first eye he wishes to examine. He tells his patient that absolutely no part of the following procedure will offer physical discomfort, and he stresses the importance of keeping the eye to be examined both wide open and unblinking. By moving the entire apparatus—tonometer, microscope, and illumination system—slightly forward, the physician is able to then slowly bring the tonometer into direct contact with his patient's cornea. When it has reached the point of proper focus, the opthalmologist will see a pair of bright yellow-green, semicircular arcs in sharp outline within his viewing scope.

The physician then adjusts the tonometer's calibrated drum until he is able to make the two fluorescent semicircles overlap; at that point, he reads the eye's intraocular pressure from a scale on the tonometer's calibrated drum. The other eye is then measured and the entire process may be repeated as often as three times until the physician has obtained a reasonably con-stant figure. These repeated efforts are often necessary for a completely accurate measurement because the initial ap-prehension that is felt by many patients who undergo tonometry may lead to an incorrectly high reading during the first or even the second attempt.

More Tests Can Be Helpful

Although the ophthalmologist may already have a pretty good idea as to whether his patient is suffering from glaucoma or not, several other tests are available to him if questions still remain. These include an examination of the patient's visual field, the *provocative test* (or *water test*), and a process called *tonography.*

Measurement of the patient's visual field is an important way to check for glaucoma because peripheral vision is the first to be affected by this disease. While a variety of sophisti-cated instruments now exist to aid the ophthalmologist in measuring peripheral vision, most utilize a central target at which the patient focuses and a controllable series of white lights that can be flashed within a hemispheric dome that sur-rounds the patient's head. By varying the size, location, and in-tensity of these lights, the physician can determine whether a loss of peripheral vision has already been experienced.

Even with all of the space-age examination equipment that is available today, there are still occasional times when glaucoma may be strongly suspected although it cannot be unquestionably diagnosed. Intraocular pressure can fluctuate, for example, and it can therefore appear normal even while the aqueous humor's outflow is restricted. In addition, the disease may not have progressed far enough to be uncovered by a visual examination of the retina and optic nerve. Still, the patient may fit the ailment's high-risk categories and complain of diminished peripheral vision.

While cases such as this are increasingly rare in this high-tech era, when they occur the ophthalmologist may use the provocative test in order to literally provoke symptoms of the disorder in his patient. This quite simple test involves the patient drinking large quantities of water over a specified period of time, during which the physician will continuously measure his intraocular pressure by means of a tonometer. Since the introduction of a large amount of water will cause the fluid that enters the patient's eyes to increase, any interference with the rate of its exit can be noted. While this test may prove helpful, it is not considered foolproof and it, too, sometimes will fail to detect glaucoma even when the disease is present.

The final common testing process, tonography, involves the physician's reading of intraocular pressure while the patient's eye is subjected to the weight of a Schiotz tonometer for several minutes. The purpose of this examination is to discover how quickly the patient's pressure will decrease under this artificial load, thereby checking his eye's ability to permit the exit of aqueous humor from the anterior chamber. The principal reason for giving this test is that tonometry alone may not provide sufficient information about the eye unless it is repeated several times during a twenty-four hour period.

THE DIFFERENT TYPES OF GLAUCOMA

Although glaucoma is generally discussed as if it were one disease, it actually consists of four commonly recognized varieties. While each develops differently, all are characterized by some type of obstruction that interferes with the aqueous humor's ability to exit from the eye. These four basic types also can be broken down into two larger categories—*primary glaucoma,* which appears without any obvious cause, and *secondary glaucoma,* which results from some other disease process or pathological condition of the eye.

Taken together, the various types of primary glaucoma are the most common forms of the disease and they are usually considered the most destructive. They also vary widely: one variety takes a long time to develop, one comes on so swiftly it may require emergency treatment, and one stems from defects in the eye's drainage system that actually were present at birth.

On the other hand, secondary glaucoma can occur at any age, in any eye, and at practically any time as a result of some other disease or disorder that has produced an obstruction in the eye's drainage system. Certain injuries, a variety of drugs, hemorrhages, tumors, and inflammations all have been known to block the channels needed for the aqueous humor to successfully exit from the inner eye. Occasionally, this variety will make itself known by resulting in some pain to the patient. While this type of glaucoma is not uncommon, it also is not the variety faced by the largest number of potential victims.

Congenital glaucoma, a primary form that is caused by a genetic predisposition to blockage or a malformation of the eye and is often present at birth, also does not present the greatest worry to most ophthalmologists and their patients. Because glaucoma in the young is relatively rare, however, increased intraocular pressure among members of this age group may go unrecognized for months or even years. So it is especially important that parents, pediatricians, and family physicians keep alert for all possible symptoms. Therefore, any obvious eye problem that is apparently suffered by an infant or young child, such as a severe sensitivity to light or excessive tearing, should be checked immediately by an ophthalmologist.

A third variety, which is somewhat common and breaks many of the rules for the disease that already have been discussed, is *acute angle-closure glaucoma.* This form develops when the eye's drainage system blocks up suddenly and rapidly, causing fluid to immediately back up and pressure to instantly increase. Unlike other types of glaucoma, a number of obvious symptoms are associated with acute angle-closure glaucoma. These include severe pain, blurred vision, the appearance of colored haloes around lights, headaches, nausea, and even vomiting.

The onset of acute angle-closure glaucoma is swift, and the sudden and severe increase in pressure that accompanies it may require emergency treatment; blindness can result in a matter of days unless the condition is relieved promptly. Some people are highly susceptible to this form of glaucoma, and for them any action that causes a wide and sudden dilation of their pupils—such as an intense emotional experience, pain, or certain drugs—can result in a drainage obstruction.

The most common form of glaucoma is also the variety

that best fits the disease's well-known reputation as a sneak thief. Called *chronic open-angle glaucoma,* this type develops slowly and quietly as the eye's drainage system becomes smaller with age and eventually clogs up. Because this form tends to progress steadily and continuously over an extended period of time, the partial blockage that results will lead to a gradual increase in intraocular pressure that must be treated before blindness results.

Most adults who suffer from glaucoma are victims of the chronic open-angle variety, which is the form that gradually destroys the patient's optic nerve and eliminates his peripheral vision without providing any obvious symptoms. This variety occurs spontaneously, with no apparent reason, and there is no known basis for its development other than genetic or hereditary factors. Usually, only a regular and complete eye examination will reveal its existence.

PROMPT TREATMENT PREVENTS BLINDNESS

The ultimate goal in treating all forms of glaucoma is, quite simply, to prevent the patient from losing his sight. Therefore, all forms of treatment are designed to lower the patient's intraocular pressure—either by increasing the ability of the aqueous humor to exit from the inner eye or by suppressing the production of this fluid, or both. Those suffering from acute angle-closure glaucoma have few options other than surgical treatment immediately upon diagnosis; patients suffering from other varieties may first receive drug therapy until the disease progresses further.

The degree to which any glaucoma patient should be treated and the form which that treatment should take depends principally upon the condition of the optic disc at the time of diagnosis. In patients who have been diagnosed early enough—especially when no cupping has occurred yet and the intraocular pressure still is relatively low—the expense and inconvenience of conventional treatment may cause both physician and patient to decide to wait, and there is nothing wrong with that. Since modern techniques and technology now

permit the properly trained ophthalmologist to detect even subtle changes that occur in the optic disc long before any
significant damage has been done, many physicians will continue to closely monitor certain patients until their pressure becomes elevated or there is a change in the appearance of the
disc.

When it is agreed that time for treatment has arrived,
several options are available. Traditionally, all forms of glaucoma (other than acute angle-closure) have been managed
almost exclusively through the use of various drugs. These medications, called *miotics* and pioneered by a French scientist
named Louis Laqueur, are designed to decrease the patient's
intraocular pressure either by aiding the exit of aqueous humor
from the eye or by decreasing the amount of this fluid that
enters in the first place.

Miotics, which are broken down by physicians into short-
acting and long-acting varieties, usually are administered as
eye drops although various combinations of pills and injections
also may be prescribed. With long and hard-to-remember generic names such as pilocarpine hydrochloride and phospholine
iodide, these drugs have been used for many years to successfully manage the disease in many patients. In addition, a new
series of promising drugs called *beta-blockers* now are available to help lower the intraocular pressure in patients who suffer
from some specific forms of the disease.

Despite its long history of use and great potential for success in certain cases, however, drug therapy for glaucoma
does not come without its problems. To be completely effective, these drugs must be taken regularly and continuously as
prescribed; for one reason or another, some patients may forget to follow through with their medication, or they may simply
ignore their physician's instructions. Even when taken as prescribed, however, several other problems with miotics have
been noted.

Although certainly not experienced by everyone who undergoes medical treatment for glaucoma, side effects and in-
tolerances to these drugs are not uncommon. A variety of unpleasant physical reactions, including headaches and blurred

vision, can serve to counterbalance the effectiveness of miotics for many patients. A sensitivity or intolerance to this type of medication, with symptoms ranging from an unpleasant drying or wrinkling of the eyelids to a serious reduction in vision, also may prohibit their use. And in some patients, their use simply may prove totally ineffective.

Surgical Options Are Available

For these reasons, as well as the immediate need to open the sudden blockage that is associated with acute angle-closure glaucoma, several forms of surgical treatment also have been developed over the years. While these methods never have been able to reverse the effects of any optic nerve destruction that already has taken place, they often are effective in preventing further vision damage. Until just a few years ago, however, state-of-the-art glaucoma surgery was inhibited severely by the lack of precision tools and techniques available to the eye surgeon. But, as in so many other areas of ophthalmology, space-age technology has changed the picture dramatically.

In the past, several relatively crude but still effective forms of surgery were performed on patients who were suffering from acute angle-closure glaucoma, as well as those who had fallen victim to other forms of the disease and did not respond properly to medical treatment. The basic goal of these procedures, which evolved from initial experiments conducted more than a century ago by Albertus von Graefe of Germany and Priestly Smith of England, was to try and stop the destruction caused by glaucoma through one of three surgical techniques.

The first of these procedures, known as an *iridectomy* or *iridotomy* and developed in the mid–nineteenth century, tries to create a more direct access to the existing drainage angle by removing a portion of the patient's iris. The second, which is called a *trabeculectomy* or *filtering operation* and was somewhat modernized in the 1960s, attempts to keep the patient's intraocular pressure within normal bounds by creating a new or improved drainage outlet for his aqueous humor. The third, which is much less common and usually performed only on older patients, involves an effort to actually decrease the patient's production of aqueous humor by the use of a tiny ice probe.

Until very recently, each one of these procedures was a completely manual operation requiring good sharp blades and a steady surgical hand. The filtering operation, for example, could be performed in several different ways but all of them involved the eye surgeon's use of a knife to create an artificial passageway through the outer wall of the patient's eye. While the resulting passageway, called a *fistula* or a *filtering bleb,* would often allow the builtup aqueous humor to again drain properly from the inner eye, the procedure was not an easy one and it sometimes led to complications of its own.

Just a few years ago, an iridectomy—which also plays an important role in today's high-tech cataract removals—was a critical but tricky procedure that was performed with the aid of a sharp knife. Although these primitive efforts often proved successful, the technique and technology available to the operating ophthalmologist at that time usually presented him with a separate but equally perplexing series of difficulties.

In the manual form of iridectomy, a tiny bit of the patient's iris is removed with a knife in order to once again allow his aqueous humor to flow properly. If performed early enough, this procedure can also prevent the iris from coming into contact with the eye's drainage area, the trabecula, and thus obstructing it. But if the patient is suffering from an acute attack of glaucoma or his iris is already adhering to the trabecula, this technique may not succeed.

Over the past few years, however, several types of laser therapy basically have replaced the outdated manual procedures that often were used to treat glaucoma in years past. Patients suffering from acute angle-closure glaucoma (which nearly always requires an operation), chronic open-angle glaucoma, and even certain types of secondary glaucoma now can be treated successfully with one of two ophthalmic lasers. These alternative procedures can be performed in short, safe, outpatient operations that most physicians consider to be even more effective than their predecessors.

Glaucoma Laser Surgery

Before proceeding with laser surgery, the ophthalmologist generally will take into account several factors in addition to the success or failure of prior medical treatment. These usually will include his patient's age and general health, the condition of the other eye, the current intraocular pressure, the appearance of the optic disc, and the existing deterioration of the visual field. If the patient is a victim of an acute glaucoma attack, however, most of these points will become secondary. The knowledge that an immediate laser operation could be the only way to save this patient's vision will really be the main factor taken into consideration.

Initially, the high-tech versions of trabeculectomy (called *laser trabeculasty*) and iridotomy both were performed exclusively with the aid of an argon laser. By utilizing this popular low-powered instrument, which many ophthalmologists already have installed right in their own offices or outpatient operating suites, the surgical techniques that are available to relieve the pressures of glaucoma immediately became simplified as well as safer and more effective.

Glaucoma patients who are selected for this noninvasive argon treatment will be brought into the outpatient operating room and then given a drop of topical anesthesia by either the ophthalmologist or an assistant. With the laser set to function in either its green or blue-green light spectrum, the eye surgeon will aim a fifty-micron spot of highly focused argon energy directly at a precise location on the patient's afflicted eye. This spot will be trained on the eye for approximately one-tenth of a second, with the laser's exact power varied according to the pigment or color that is present within the patient's ocular structures.

The ophthalmologist who is performing an argon-laser trabeculoplasty will place several "burns" on the angle of his patient's eye that has become clogged and impeded the exit of aqueous humor. It is believed that by using a laser to *photo-coagulate* these blocked pores, they will then open up and once more allow this fluid to flow naturally. The eye surgeon who is performing a laser iridotomy will use the argon to literally drill a tiny opening in a part of his patient's iris, thus permitting the aqueous humor to circulate freely again and the intraocular pressure to decrease.

The Latest Laser Option

Even more recently, however, an additional innovation has been brought to glaucoma surgery. Today, many ophthalmologists are switching from the argon to the newer neodymium-YAG laser for angle-closure glaucoma treatment as well as for the management of several other eye disorders. Because of its ability to penetrate very deeply within human tissue and stop the bleeding in large blood vessels, the YAG was first used medically on those patients who were hemorrhaging from stomach ulcers; it was later used to combat the early stages of bladder cancer. Eye surgeons quickly spotted its potential and rapidly employed the YAG for their precision ocular work.

While the various glaucoma-management procedures that are performed with the aid of an argon or a YAG laser may seem quite similar to the patient, there are in fact several significant differences. Glaucoma patients who are about to undergo a YAG laser treatment will be given a drop of topical anesthesia and then seated before the eye surgeon's slit lamp. After they receive a full explanation of the short outpatient procedure they are about to undergo, a weak aiming beam of helium-neon laser light will be shined directly into their afflicted eye.

The ophthalmologist utilizes this aiming beam to accurately select the proper location for focusing his powerful YAG beam; depending upon the exact procedure he has scheduled, he then will fire from two to five bursts of the YAG laser in order to open a blocked angle by drilling a small hole in the patient's iris. Almost immediately after the procedure, the patient will leave the ophthalmologist's office with instructions to use prescribed eye drops for one week together with any other anti-glaucoma medications that may be needed.

CONTINUED ATTENTION IS VITALLY IMPORTANT

Treatments performed with the YAG laser offer great promise for many glaucoma patients, and this newer device can even be used to reopen an argon laser iridotomy that has become blocked with pigment following the initial surgery. Still, it must always be remembered that laser therapy does not actually *cure* the patient's glaucoma. It may stabilize the disease and prevent any additional loss of vision, and it may substantially reduce the amount of antiglaucoma medication that the patient is required to take, or even liberate him entirely from these drugs. For the rest of their lives, however, all patients who have suffered from glaucoma, regardless of the treatment they have received, must continue to undergo periodic examinations for any signs that the disease has resumed its destructive path.

This is not to suggest that all glaucoma patients must shut themselves off immediately from the world and then totally readjust their lifestyles. On the contrary, thanks to the wide variety of medical and surgical treatments that are available today, glaucoma patients do not have to restrict their work schedules or other activities at all. Exercise programs need not be given up, and some ophthalmologists believe that a vigorous workout may even slightly lower the patient's intraocular pressure for short periods. Reasonable food and drink intake also has no known effect on the disease (although a large volume of water consumed during a short time *can* increase the eye's internal pressure). Even the ingestion of coffee, tea, or alcohol is not known to produce any detrimental effects.

Still, the continuation of regular checkups is crucial because glaucoma can worsen or improve suddenly without the patient even being aware that his condition has altered. These subtle changes may require a shift in treatment, however, and so the patient's physician must remain constantly in touch with the situation. It is critically important, therefore, that both patient and ophthalmologist work together to keep this disease under control.

One way to do that is for those who have been diagnosed previously as well as those who are in the prime age and risk groups to remain aware of any symptoms that might appear. A gradual but progressive shrinking of the peripheral or side vision, while often difficult to detect, may be noticed by some patients and should always lead immediately to a visit to an ophthalmologist. Blurred vision and colored haloes around lights may also signal the onset of glaucoma; if these signs are accompanied by nausea and vomiting, a physician should be consulted immediately.

Pain in the eye, of course, is a sign of trouble that should never be ignored. Although the most common form of glaucoma (open-angle) may progress to total blindness without any accompanying physical discomfort whatsoever, pain usually is experienced by victims of angle-closure glaucoma as well as those who suffer from some of the other less common varieties of the disease. While the reason for this inconsistency is not entirely clear, it appears as if pain in glaucoma is related to the rapidity of increase in intraocular pressure—the faster this tension builds, the more pain will be experienced.

REGULAR EXAMS ARE CRITICAL

If all forms of glaucoma offered us such clear and distinct symptoms, the available treatment for its effects could be utilized more effectively. Unfortunately, it is the most common form of glaucoma that provides us with few clues to its existence; and young people unaware of this or any other disease are susceptible to its destruction. Thorough eye examinations, therefore, remain the best way to catch the disorder before its damage becomes too severe.

Infants and children, who obviously cannot be expected to monitor themselves, should be examined for glaucoma and other eye disorders immediately upon the detection of any overt signs or symptoms. Newborn infants with a high risk of glaucoma and infantile cataracts, such as those with a family history of either disease, should be given an ophthalmological exam even before they are discharged from the hospital nursery. Older children who have not exhibited any obvious problems with their eyesight still should be examined by age three or four to check for the presence of ocular disorders as well as to measure their visual acuity. Regular screenings of all school-age children should be undertaken approximately once every two years.

Although we as adults should know better, many of us simply "forget" to schedule appointments with our eye doctors until an obvious problem has arisen. Fortunately, for a large portion of our adult lives this can be viewed as entirely acceptable behavior. It is commonly recognized these days that, following puberty, there will usually be little change in a patient's existing refractive error. Additionally, any significant development of eye disease also tends to be low at this time. Healthy adults under age forty, therefore, do not need to have their eyes checked very often in the absence of overt symptoms or vision problems.

Despite any prior habits that we have developed, however, all of us should begin a series of regular eye exams once we pass age forty. From then on, we should visit an ophthalmologist every two to five years for a thorough glaucoma evaluation. For those of us who fit into any of the disease's high-risk categories, the period between these checkups will usually be much shorter and should be determined by an eye physician.

These important examinations are quick and painless, and even those of us who cannot afford to visit a private physician in his office usually can obtain a public-clinic screening within our communities. Often provided at minimal or even no cost, these large-scale screenings for visual disorders (including glaucoma) are staged regularly by volunteer civic organizations, religious groups, community centers, nursing homes, hospitals, and private-practice ophthalmologists. Although results from busy screenings may not always prove completely accurate, they will provide most participants with an indication of existing problems and introduce them to professionals who can offer further help.

Space-age technology and modern ophthalmic technique have permitted eye surgeons to make great strides in their ongoing battle against glaucoma. Once this troublesome eye disorder has been detected, therefore, today's ophthalmology can provide tremendous hope to its victims. Since the disease will rarely reveal itself until long after its destructive process is underway, it still remains up to the patient to nip glaucoma's damage in the bud.

6

The Battle Against Retinal

Disorders

If any of us were asked to name the one part of the eye that we consider to be most responsible for vision, we would be faced with a difficult task. As previous chapters in this book have described, all these incredibly tiny parts have their own specific and important roles. All are superb examples of perfection in miniaturization and specialization and they must all work together as a smoothly functioning team in order for clear eyesight to result.

Each of the eye's individual components is so integral to the process of human vision, in fact, we probably could make a pretty good case for practically every single part. The cornea and the lens are both vital focusing aids that are necessary to refract incoming light rays. The aqueous humor and the vitreous humor are needed to help keep all other parts aligned and in their correct positions. The iris, ciliary body, and sclera each have their own specific and important jobs. The retina translates refracted light rays into readable signals of energy. The optic

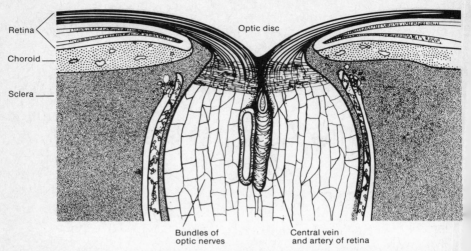

Retina

Choroid

Sclera

Optic disc

Bundles of   Central vein
optic nerves   and artery of retina

The retina performs the final step in the complex process of refraction before sending light rays through the optic nerve and on to the brain.

nerve transmits these energy signals to the brain. And so on and so on.

If continually pressed to name just *one* part, however, we might do well to select the retina. This is, after all, the final point that light rays reach during the eye's beautifully complex process of refraction. And, as we now know, without a properly functioning retina no focused images could be sent to the brain.

Despite the retina's importance, unfortunately, it is not immune to an occasional malady or disorder. Like other parts of the eye, the retina also can be stricken by destructive injuries and diseases. If this occurs, the images that it ultimately transmits to the brain will serve only as poor representations of the signals it has received. But space-age ophthalmic tools and techniques have provided today's eye surgeons with a variety of exciting new ways to patch up many of these retinal problems.

THE EYE'S "BUSINESS END"

Only about one-fiftieth of an inch thick, the retina, often called the "business end" of the eye, is a delicate, paper-thin membrane that is located between the vitreous humor and the choroid. It lines the inside of the eyeball like a curved movie screen or a cup and it covers all of the inner surface of the eyes, except the very front part where light rays first enter. The retina itself looks somewhat like a pink net and its name actually was derived from the Latin word for net, *rete*.

Among its other parts, the retina consists of an expansion of the optic nerve that allows it to serve as the eye's direct link with the brain. When refracted light rays travel through the eyeball and eventually hit the retina, they are upside down and flat; the retina's photoreceptors then convert this light into partly electrical, partly chemical signals that can be understood by the brain. These signals are passed along to the brain by way of the optic nerve, thus permitting us to visualize the images of all objects that are present before our eyes.

Although the retina's appearance is often compared to that of a movie screen, most of us would be extremely unhappy to be seated in a theater with a screen that is just like a retina. Unlike a (usually) flawless movie screen, for example, the retina is composed of various veins and arteries that provide it with areas of greater and lesser sensitivity. Our acute vision, therefore, functions only with objects that are viewed directly in front of us and whose refracted images can fall on a tiny pit in the center of the retina called the *fovea;* another 1.5-centimeter spot, where the optic nerve fibers leave the eye, has no light-responsive cells at all and is literally blind. A movie screen that contained such obvious faults would have the entire theater audience up and screaming for the manager.

When it comes to the retina, however, these "imperfections" are part of the whole design. The primary destination of all light rays that reach the retina is a group of some 130 million light-sensitive cells at its back known as *rods* and *cones*. The cones, concentrated on the central fovea, are for color and daylight vision and are capable of producing the clearest signals to be sent to the brain. The rods, which are predominant outside the fovea, are for black-and-white and night vision. Working together, the rods and cones produce the kind of clear and effortless eyesight that we have come to expect.

Problems Do Develop

These important parts of the retina can break down, though, and when that happens a variety of disorders can result. Some, such as the so-called *rod syndromes* and *cone syndromes,* are relatively minor. Their existence primarily requires the patient who suffers from them to undergo a series of mental adjustments in order to compensate for the inconveniences that they may cause.

These two minor disorders relate primarily to inadequacies in the retinal parts that bear their names and they generally show up as malfunctions in the jobs that these parts are intended to perform. Cone syndromes, for example, frequently result in color blindness, somewhat decreased visual acuity, and decreased vision in bright light. Rod syndromes, on the other hand, usually are characterized by an inability to see well at night (commonly known as *night blindness*) or a difficulty in adjusting well to dim light. None of these deficiencies are sight-threatening, and nearly all of those who experience them will be able to continue to lead perfectly normal lives.

There are, however, a series of much more serious disorders that can strike the retina and threaten its ability to function correctly. It is therefore important that these ailments, which include *macular degeneration, retinal detachment,* and *retinopathy,* be diagnosed as soon as possible because they usually will require immediate ophthalmic care. If left untreated, these problems will lead to almost certain vision impairment and they may even result in total blindness.

Fortunately, today's ophthalmology has introduced several new and effective methods that have proven useful in diagnosing and treating a number of these more serious retinal disorders. High-tech instruments that allow the ophthalmologist to see all the way through the eye to the retina have aided in the initial discovery of these ailments; lasers and other instruments have helped in their eventual treatment. Many retinal problems that regularly resulted in blindness in the past, in fact, now can be uncovered and treated well before a loss of vision occurs.

COMPLETE EXAM IS CRITICAL

Like so many other vision disorders, a complete examination by a qualified ophthalmologist is critical to the proper diagnosis and treatment of these ailments, and an exam should be scheduled as soon as possible after any symptoms are noticed. The signs that are most commonly associated with retinal disorders are so-called *flashes* and *floaters*, and when they are detected a physician should be consulted immediately. However, a variety of other symptoms may also signal the onset of a retinal problem—including decreased vision, the presence of certain diseases, the feeling that a hazy curtain is hanging in front of the eye, or the perception that a "smudge" is obscuring some portions of the visual field—and these should lead to an eye exam as well.

At an examination for the detection of a possible retinal disorder, the ophthalmologist will first ask several questions to help him narrow down the scope of potential problems. He will inquire as to whether the symptoms appeared suddenly or gradually (sudden symptoms could mean a retinal problem while gradual symptoms may mean a cataract), and he will ask about the patient's general health (diabetes and hypertension can affect the retina).

The physician will then begin to examine his patient's retina. After dilating his pupils, he usually will start by looking through an ophthalmoscope. This hand-held instrument can be focused on the back of the patient's eye unless a cataract is present. If no cataract is found, however, the opthalmologist may assume that his patient's problem does indeed stem from a retinal ailment. He then will begin to specifically diagnose which of a variety of problems it may be.

Macular Degeneration Is Least Serious

Probably the least serious of all the major retinal disorders, but one that requires immediate attention nonetheless, is a disease called macular degeneration. While this condition can strike practically anyone and may be hereditary or result from some other disease, it seems to occur most often among those of advanced age. Fortunately, macular degeneration almost never leads to total blindness, although it can dramatically affect the patient's central reading vision.

The macula is the name for the tiny center of the retina that is responsible for most of what we ultimately see. As we age, however, it degenerates naturally, in part due to changes in the eye's blood supply that lead to alternations in the blood vasculature. The resulting breakdown can lead to a gradual loss of central vision, which is referred to as *dry macular degeneration;* for those afflicted with so-called *wet macular degeneration,* blindness can result.

Retinal changes of this type often begin with a series of small hemorrhages in the macular area. These may be followed by pigmentary disturbances that appear to the ophthalmologist in the form of yellowish spots with irregular black stippling. In the course of a thorough retinal examination, the physician may also see a deep-red, round, punched-out patch with clean-cut grayish edges situated at the macula. This is a so-called *hole in the macula* and will clearly signal the presence of macular degeneration.

Most patients who exhibit these symptoms will then be evaluated further with the use of a space-age photographic technique called *fluorescein angiography.* This permits the physician to search more closely for the existence and location of any abnormal blood vessels that might be present. Once they are uncovered by this modern procedure, these abnormal blood vessels can be destroyed before additional hemorrhaging or scarring can affect the patient's central vision.

Help Is Available

In the past, one of the only treatments for macular degeneration was a strong warning that the patient stay out of the sun entirely, or else venture outdoors only when wearing a pair of sophisticated, ultraviolet-absorbing sunglasses. It has long been recognized that continuous doses of powerful ultraviolet light, such as that found in most parts of the southwestern United States, can cause certain people to develop these degenerative changes. So it naturally followed that a lack of sunlight or the application of ultraviolet-absorbing sunglasses could be somewhat successful in preventing further deterioration of the central retina. And often, it was.

It was not until the recent development of ophthalmic laser surgery, however, that a real treatment could be developed for this troublesome disorder. Today, certain patients suffering from macular degeneration can be treated in an office setting with an argon or krypton laser, which are so accurate that they can be used to actually destroy these abnormal blood vessels. Unfortunately, most patients who already have experienced a deterioration of the central retina usually cannot benefit from this type of laser therapy. But for others, these high-tech tools can offer a safe and effective alternative to the internal destruction and vision impairment that macular degeneration ultimately can cause.

As is the case with so many ophthalmic disorders, treat-

This Amsler Grid will allow a patient to test himself for the presence of macular degeneration by following the simple instructions included in the text.

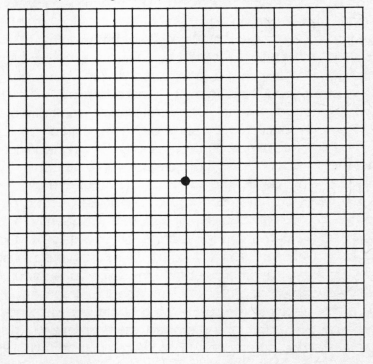

ment for macular degeneration is most effective when the disease is detected early. An actual diagnosis can only be made by an ophthalmologist after a thorough examination, of course, but a simple at-home test can help any patient to determine the possibility of the disease's presence and thus lead to a timely eye exam.

To test yourself for macular degeneration, place the Amsler grid illustrated here on any bare wall or door in a well-lighted room so that the central dot on the chart appears at eye level. Next, mark off a spot on the floor that is fourteen inches from the chart and stand facing the grid with your heels on the spot you have marked. Wearing your eyeglasses only if they are prescribed for reading, look at the dot while covering your left eye; then look at the dot while covering your right eye. If the grid appears to be blurry or has any blank spots, a visit to the ophthalmologist is in order.

Retinal Detachment Is a Serious Problem

Another related problem, for which high-tech tools and techniques have proven effective, is retinal detachment. Forty years ago, a diagnosis of retinal detachment almost always meant that the patient would become blind in the afflicted eye; surgery sometimes was attempted, but the cure rate generally was only about one in every hundred cases. Today, however, the introduction and successful use of ophthalmic laser treatment—which allows the modern eye surgeon to "spot-weld" the tiny retinal rips and tears that later can lead to total detachment—has boosted that cure rate to 95 percent.

While retinal detachment remains a serious eye problem, it is no longer as common a cause of blindness as cataracts or even glaucoma. The disorder occurs most frequently in those over age fifty, and many physicians believe it is most often found among those aged fifty to sixty. It is discovered in about two out of every hundred people in the target age group, with the largest percentage of its victims also found to be suffering from nearsightedness (because the myopic eye is elongated these retinas already are stretched and therefore have the greatest chance of developing a tear). Additionally, the problem can result from a blow to the eye, a cyst or a tumor, scar tissue, a hemorrhage, an infection or some other eye disease, and even a general tendency toward poor retinal adhesion.

The primary symptom of a torn retina—called *flashes and floaters*—usually is seen in only one eye but nevertheless can appear to the patient in a variety of ways. It may start as a sudden flash of light in the lower part of her visual field. It may develop as a shower of spots that continually rains in front of her affected eye. It may look like small dots or wiggly lines that appear to float within her field of vision. It may even show up as a hazy curtain before the afflicted eye or an unexplained drop in that eye's visual acuity.

If any of these flashes or floaters do develop, it is very important for the patient to see an ophthalmologist within a day or so of their onset. Most people will experience such symptoms at some point in their lives and their development does not definitely mean that the patient's retina already has become detached. However, their appearance does suggest that the problem could be in its early stages and, as with most other common eye disorders, early diagnosis is the key to successful treatment.

Despite the variety of specific causes, a retinal tear usually develops in one of two basic ways. The first is a natural part of aging, and stems from the eye's vitreous humor first adhering to the retina and then shrinking in quantity. If this occurs, the vitreous humor may actually pull the retina away from its adjoining layer, known as the choroid, and eventually result in a retinal detachment.

The second way may be more common, however, because it comes after some type of hole or tear has initially appeared in the patient's retina. Once these holes or tears have developed, a small amount of vitreous humor, which often changes from its original jellylike consistency to a liquified substance during the aging process, may begin to seep through them and force its way behind the retina. If the vitreous humor manages to fill the space between the retina and the choroid, it may also cause these two loosely attached layers to begin to separate. In the absence of proper care, the retina and choroid will peel away from each other completely and a detached retina will result.

Treatment Follows A Full Exam

Whatever the disorder's origin, without prompt treatment it certainly can prove to be a very serious problem. Since the choroid contains the blood vessels that nourish the retina and its millions of nerve cells, a separation of these two layers will reduce the retina's essential blood supply and prevent this critical part of the eye from properly doing its job. If the detachment grows complete and the blood supply is totally cut off, the retina will become useless and blindness will result. Despite years of research, surgery remains the only known cure for the problem of retinal detachment.

When symptoms like flashes and floaters have been detected and a visit to the ophthalmologist has been scheduled, a thorough examination with today's high-tech tools can help to pinpoint the precise problem. A detached retina usually is diagnosed with the aid of an ophthalmoscope, which actually can allow the physician to see the exact point of separation between retina and choroid. If an examination is undertaken early enough, it also can permit him to see any holes or tears that exist and will be likely to precede the more serious end result.

The first successful treatment for retinal detachment was developed back in 1919 by a Swiss doctor named Jules Gronin. After studying the troublesome problem and its apparent cause quite extensively, Gronin suggested that a process called *thermocautery,* in which an adhesive scar is burned around the point of separation and then used to reattach the two layers, might prove effective. A period of widespread experimentation did show that this daring form of cauterization therapy was somewhat helpful, as was another early method of care occasionally attempted at the time that utilized an ice probe to literally freeze the two separated layers into reattachment known as *cryosurgery.*

Although these treatment measures quickly gained some

favor among pioneer ophthalmologists because they were recognizably better than anything known before, the day's early ophthalmic tools made the procedures almost prohibitively difficult to perform. Eye surgeons lacked a way to accurately view the retinal area in which they were operating, for example, and they lacked the fine instruments necessary to work within such a tiny area. The cure rate for retinal detachment still hovered around the unacceptable rate of one percent, and its diagnosis justifiably would send shivers of concern down the spines of its victims.

THE LASER WAS THE TURNING POINT

As with so many other eye ailments, however, the turning point that put an end to this disorder's destructive cycle also arrived with the development and perfection of the argon laser. Used promptly after the initial discovery of any holes or tears in the patient's retina, the argon beam actually can stop a detachment from occurring. Its effectiveness has been so remarkable, in fact, that many believe it is almost singlehandedly responsible for the rapid decline in blindness that previously was associated with this once-dreaded eye problem.

Utilizing the accuracy that only a laser can provide, in conjunction with the remarkable viewing power of today's operating microscopes, the ophthalmologist treating a retinal tear can now see what he is doing and do what he sees is needed. In a short, safe, and effective outpatient operation, he can aim an argon beam directly through his patient's pupil and use its power to coagulate most holes or tears that exist long before they can result in a complete retinal detachment. If a detachment already has occurred, however, he may have to resort to additional surgical procedures to treat the patient.

Still, even with the great promises that stem from today's argon procedure, the success rate for this space-age technique is only 95 percent. ("Success" is considered to be a retina that remains attached and vision that remains totally unimpaired.) This lack of absolute perfection comes from the disorder's initially hard-to-read development. Despite what appears to be a successful treatment by ophthalmic laser, for example, some damage to the eye's retinal tissue may have been suffered even before a proper diagnosis was made, and a degree of vision loss already may have occurred. Even with a perfect laser coagulation, therefore, the treatment may not be deemed a "success."

The amount of vision impairment that can result from this eye disorder also depends upon the exact point at which the retinal separation originally has taken place. If the detachment occurs on the retina's periphery, little or no vision loss will result; if it occurs close to the retina's center, a possibility of far greater vision impairment must be expected. But no matter where detachment occurs, once it does, the retinal tissue at that spot will no longer function and some sight will be lost.

When undertaken in time, today's high-tech treatment for retinal detachment can help to prevent most vision loss. Once again, however, the key to success still is prompt diagnosis, preferably before any holes or tears have had a chance to cause an actual separation. Only then can the ophthalmologist utilize his tools and techniques to their full advantage.

Retinopathy Is a Major Cause of Blindness

Another major cause of blindness that is related to the retina is a very serious disease called retinopathy. This is an abnormal and relatively uncommon condition that is usually marked by a variety of degenerative changes occuring within the patient's retina, often involving a breakdown in its structure, chemistry, or circulation. There also are two basic and quite different forms of this ailment, which usually develops as a by-product of either diabetes or hypertension.

Retinopathy of hypertension actually is the least worrisome of the disease's two types, even though it can prove to be equally destructive if left untreated. In this form, the eye's *arterioles* (which are the smallest of the arteries that bring blood to the capillaries) become constricted. The small vessels supplying blood to the retina grow deformed, some burst, and hemorrhages can occur. If left untreated, this condition may result in a total loss of the patient's critical central vision.

Although potential damage from this form of retinopathy can be very severe, blindness actually will result from it only on very rare occasions. This is because a hypertension problem that is serious enough to cause the eye disorder more than likely will lead to the patient's death well before such total visual destruction has occurred. Retinopathy of hypertension can be successfully controlled by managing the patient's high blood pressure.

Diabetic retinopathy, on the other hand, is potentially a much more serious problem because it affects a great number of those who suffer from diabetes and it must be treated on its own. New high-tech therapies to combat the disorder have been developed in recent years, but since the discovery of insulin more and more diabetics are living longer lives—which ironically also gives them more time to develop related problems like diabetic retinopathy. Despite the exciting new treatments that are available, therefore, this disease still has become one of the leading causes of new blindness throughout the world and some 45 percent of all diabetics eventually will lose their vision because of it.

Diabetes is a common disorder whose diagnosed victims number about one-and-a-half percent of the Western world's population. The number of as-yet undetected cases, however, is believed to boost this percentage closer to five percent. It is also estimated that in the United States alone there are a total of approximately 4 million diagnosed and as-yet undetected cases, with about 150,000 new patients uncovered each year. Additionally, diabetes occurs slightly more often among females than among males, and some 50 percent of all cases first develop in those aged forty to fifty.

The incidence of diabetic retinopathy varies directly with the age of onset of diabetes and with the length of time the disease has been present. For example, diabetic retinopathy can be expected to develop in fully 90 percent of all those who have suffered from diabetes for more than eighteen years. With a few rare exceptions, all diabetics who have had the disease for more than twenty-five years will be expected to show some signs of the eye disorder.

Diabetic Retinopathy Has Only Recently Been Understood

The overall problem of diabetic retinopathy and its relation to diabetes could not be studied satisfactorily until 1962, for it was not until that year that researchers first learned that diabetic dogs often developed a similar eye disorder. After two decades of study, the major factor in the eye problem's origination now is thought to be circulatory-related because diabetes produces abnormalities such as aneurysms in the tiny blood vessels that deliver arterial blood to the retina and pick up waste products for removal through the veins. Researchers have determined that diabetics who experience circulatory damage also suffer from an interference in their system's ability to deliver nutrients and remove waste from cells and nerves of the retina.

Today, the term *diabetic retinopathy* usually is applied to a group of changes that occur in the eye of a diabetic patient. These changes generally consist of hemorrhages, blood vessel alterations, and microaneurysms, the most serious of which involves the formation of new blood vessels. The ailment comes in a variety of forms, ranging from a mild condition with no symptoms to a severe and irreversible disease. The disease is so varied, in fact, that no two eyes diagnosed with diabetic retinopathy will show exactly the same condition and development.

Although it is usually referred to as one disease, diabetic retinopathy actually has been subdivided into two categories. One, called *proliferative retinopathy*, is marked by the growth of new blood vessels on the surface of the retina which may at some point lead to scarring and hemorrhaging. The other, known as *edematous* or *background retinopathy*, is characterized by the leakage of small blood vessels that ultimately may result in diminished vision. Despite the knowledge that has been gained about both forms of diabetic retinopathy in recent years, however, the evolution of these two categories is so variable that neither is yet completely understood.

Those who suffer from diabetic retinopathy may not experience any vision impairment at all in the disorder's early stages, so a regular eye examination is particularly important for those who have suffered from diabetes for a number of years. While some forms of the eye disease are not diagnosed until it is too late to stop its destruction, today's ophthalmic technology and techniques have opened up a variety of exciting new options for many others.

Initial Treatments Were Ineffective

Before high technology was introduced to the world of eye surgery, however, this was not usually the case. A variety of diverse medical efforts which scientists believed might be useful in treating diabetic retinopathy have appeared on the scene almost constantly since World War II, but every single one of them has eventually proved to be ineffective. Most, in fact, were discarded almost immediately after a brief period of unsuccessful experimentation.

In conjunction with the ongoing knowledge that physicians have been gaining over the years about the onset of diabetes itself, various regimens to prevent the initial development of retinopathy—including diet management and insulin administration—have also been tried. However, none of these attempts, as well as related efforts to control the specific amount of carbohydrates, proteins, and fats that diabetics ingest, have proven successful in halting retinopathy's spread.

Since the 1950s, physicians also have introduced a number of programs that were aimed at reversing the various cases of diabetic retinopathy that already had been diagnosed. These optimistic efforts have included special diets; the use of food supplements and vitamins; the prescription of drugs that affect blood lipids; the development of various plans that utilize anticoagulants, hormones, and anabolic steroids; and even X-ray therapy. Nonetheless, despite a concerted effort on the part of the medical community, all of them have proven completely negative or, at best, have offered only a very limited usefulness.

The first successful surgical attempt to halt the certain visual destruction of diabetic retinopathy was the use of a procedure called *hypophysectomy*. This technique, which is usually performed by someone other than an eye surgeon, involves the removal of all or a part of the patient's pituitary gland. Although this method of treatment is utilized only rarely today, it did prove somewhat useful before the development of modern space-age ophthalmic tools rendered it out of date.

LASERS OFFER NEW OPTIONS

The initial high-tech attack on diabetic retinopathy was made with the aid of a xenon arc, which is an early ophthalmic laser that first enabled eye surgeons to photocoagulate and destroy many of the disease-related abnormal blood vessels and aneurysms on an outpatient basis. Used primarily in cases of retinopathy in which a vitreous hemorrhage already had occurred, the intense white light of the xenon arc could be focused on the retina following dilation of the pupil and a simple retrobulbar injection for pain control. The surgeon could then burn away the diseased bodies in a matter of seconds.

Unfortunately, despite its occasional effectiveness, a xenon-arc treatment alone often did not end every patient's bout with retinopathy. The xenon cannot, for example, successfully destroy any abnormal blood vessels that are elevated above the surface of the retina. It also proves ineffective with blood vessels that are located directly on the optic nerve head. For these and certain other cases, an argon-laser treatment may be required.

For retinal work, just as it has done in other ophthalmic applications, the argon laser quickly has proven itself to be a marvelously effective and almost invaluable tool. Since it can photocoagulate blood vessels using only one-fifth of the energy required by a white xenon arc, its related increase in efficiency is obvious. Since it can operate accurately in spots only one-fifth the size necessary for the use of a xenon beam, its related increase in safety cannot be understated.

Not long after its introduction into the ophthalmic community, it quickly became apparent that the argon laser would work very well within the close and intricate confines of the eye's retina. After being used initially in cooperation with the xenon arc in order to treat certain cases of retinopathy, the argon laser rapidly came into its own as an effective and safe outpatient laser treatment for nearly all instances of the disease. As soon as it became readily available to most ophthalmologists, the argon laser was recognized as the definitive tool of choice for most physicians who practice retinal surgery.

Space-age ophthalmology does not stand still and the development of an even newer instrument is showing definite signs of replacing the argon laser in the treatment of diabetic retinopathy. Known as the *dye laser,* this brand-new device actually involves two lasers—an argon and a krypton—whose light beams are focused together through a dye that alters their color spectrums. Since the retina responds differently to various laser beam colors, in the future this incredible instrument also may prove helpful in treating other retinal problems with a higher degree of accuracy than has ever been possible before.

A Problem Among Premies

One final retinal problem that also is being treated with today's space-age tools and techniques requires the final word, even though it is a highly uncommon disorder that only strikes a very specific patient base. This disease is quite serious and can lead to severe complications, however, and it should be discussed because its successful treatment truly stems from the incredible high-tech advances that ophthalmologists have made in recent years. Without them, this disorder, too, can lead to dramatic vision impairment and even blindness.

The disease is known as *acute retinopathy of prematurity,* or *ROP,* and it is a retinovascular disorder found among certain

premature babies. The further back in the eye the disease is located, the younger the preterm, and the greater the amount of
tissue that is involved, the more serious the ROP can be. Generally, only the very smallest and very sickest of premature babies develop ROP. And for them, the disease can produce a
real problem.

Also called *retrolental fibroplasia,* this eye disorder was first
described by physicians in 1942. Once researchers learned during the next decade that the administration of oxygen appeared to lead to its development, the use of oxygen in incu-
bators was curtailed and the incidence of ROP dropped off. A
new epidemic surfaced in the 1970s, however, when scientific
advances made the survival of very-low-birth-weight babies a
routine occurence; unfortunately, oxygen was needed to save
these babies and oxygen still caused ROP.

Several methods of medical treatment were tried initially—including the use of Vitamin E to protect the retina during oxygen administration—but not one single effort was found
that could stop the spread of the disease. Physicians knew that
something had to be done because, if left unchecked, ROP
rapidly can progress to retinal detachment and it also can
lead to a variety of other eye problems that will cause serious
woes for the premature infant. Still, nothing seemed to work until eye surgeons turned to a pair of modified space-age
ophthalmic techniques that they usually used only on older patients.

High-Tech Treatments Adapted

After several years of experimentation it was determined in
the mid-1970s that the two procedures—cryotherapy and
photocoagulation—could be adapted successfully to the eye
of a tiny infant. If the disease is severe and its progression appears rapid, in fact, either of these two high-tech surgical procedures can be performed on an infant with ROP at twelve
weeks of age or even less. Both procedures can be performed
in a hospital's operating room, not far from the nursery in which
the baby is being watched. Both can also be performed with

the infant reclining on a warm mattress that has been placed directly upon the operating table.

In ROP cryotherapy, the baby is brought into the operating room still snug in his incubator and his pupils are dilated while an anesthesiologist is standing by to monitor all vital signs. Local anesthetic is administered by means of eyedrops, and a *baby lid speculum* is inserted to keep the infant's eyelids separated. An indirect ophthalmoscope then is moved into position in order for the eye surgeon to constantly monitor the position of his cryoprobe.

As the cryoprobe is applied, it is used to literally freeze a specific area in the baby's eye that has been preselected by a combination of knowledge about the patient's specific condition and past experience. The entire procedure takes a relatively short period of time, and a minor regimen of postoperative care includes dilating drops given daily for several weeks and the use of lightweight ice compresses to decrease local eyelid swelling. Improvement in the baby's condition can be expected within twelve to twenty-four hours and it will continue through the next two weeks, after which time the eye should be practically normal.

For some patients, photocoagulation is considered to be a more effective means of treating ROP. While this therapy only can be employed in certain cases, in these instances the argon laser has become the ophthalmic tool of choice. This procedure is usually performed under general anesthesia, and the photocoagulation is delivered by an argon beam that is trained on the patient's eye for only one- to two-tenths of a second. Postoperative care requirements are minimal after this form of treatment, too, and rapid and continued improvement is also expected.

Without a doubt, the retina is certainly a wonderful piece of machinery. By translating refracted light rays into a form that can be understood by the brain, it serves as the direct link between incoming visual messages and sight. There can be little argument, in fact, that without a retina our eyes simply could not function in the manner to which we have become accustomed.

Like other parts of the eye that work together to create vision, however, the retina also can fall victim to a variety of ailments and disorders that will minimize its effectiveness. Without proper treatment, these various retinal problems can lead to diminished vision or even blindness. Since these diseases often come with little or no warning, their damage, once done, is oftentimes irreversible.

Fortunately, modern ophthalmology has developed a number of high-tech tools and techniques that can be used to successfully combat most of these retinal disorders before their destruction has become irreparable. Lasers, cryoprobes, ophthalmoscopes, and the rest, however, can only work properly if they are used in time.

Regular, thorough eye examinations are one way that we can monitor our ocular health. A total awareness of the numerous symptoms that are related to various retinal problems is another. Taken together, examinations and awareness are the only certain ways to ensure the continued operation of the retina, our eye's most magnificent single part.

7

Vision Myths and Eye-Care

Misconceptions

Over the years, the enigmatic nature of vision and the eye has given rise to a variety of legendary myths concerned with everything from bizarre eating habits to associated supernatural powers. Most of these misbeliefs have disappeared over time, although some of the more creative ones have lingered to this day.

On the contemporary front, the fast-moving ophthalmic developments of recent decades have also been responsible for their share of wild misconceptions. Some of these, too, have been quickly forgotten while others continue to build on misinformed media reports and ill-advised gossip.

Whether such incorrect medical information is centuries-old or newly conceived, however, much the same problem can result. Although these myths are often harmless in nature, some erroneous opinions on health care in general or eye care in particular can lead to unfortunate consequences. A few can even cause patients to reject the very treatments and care that could help them to save their sight.

MISINFORMATION IS WIDESPREAD

Despite today's highly sophisticated system of mass communication, some medical information just does not make it to the public without distortion. A mid-1980s survey of Californians over the age of fifty-five, for example, showed that nearly three-quarters of the respondents believed that cataracts result from a film covering the eye and that good nutrition alone can be useful in preventing eye disease. Half of the respondents also felt that the body will sometimes reject an intraocular lens implant (IOL) and that eye surgery is safest when it is performed in a traditional hospital setting.

On one hand, these incorrect assumptions indicate that many respondents were at least somewhat aware of various developments in modern ophthalmology. On the other hand, they prove that vision myths and eye-care misconceptions develop easily and are then hard to dispel.

Part of the problem stems directly from the new technology. Quite understandably, many patients who grew up in an age before computers and satellites cannot comprehend the very concept of ophthalmic lasers and cryolathes. To them, all of the space-age equipment that is now used in eye surgery is as mysterious as space flight.

Another part of the problem comes from the new techniques. Today's high-tech procedures, after all, even confuse some physicians who do not work with them on a regular basis. How, then, can a patient, already under stress because of an eye problem, be expected to fully understand the relatively new operation that he is about to undergo?

A final part of the problem results from the eye itself. Despite the vast amount of knowledge that we have gained about it over the past forty years, certain aspects of vision still are not completely understood, even by experts.

It is therefore not surprising to learn that a number of myths continue to surround the eyes and the process of vision. In fact, most aspects of eye care—cataracts and the methods used to extract them, lasers and their surgical possibilities, refractive errors and their means of correction, contact lenses and IOLs—are the subject of quite a few mistaken beliefs.

Many of the misconceptions related to these issues have arisen simply because no single authoritative source previously existed to explain them. Patients can dispel some of this misinformation by reading the facts as they are described below; ophthalmologists who are asked direct questions can clear up other problems and concerns.

GENERAL MYTHS ABOUT EYE SURGERY

Myth #1: Surgery of the eye, especially using the new tools and techniques, is quite painful and recovery time will be lengthy.

Fact: Actually, patients who undergo most of today's high-tech ophthalmic surgical procedures will experience relatively little pain, if any at all. The space-age techniques described in this book are almost always performed under local anesthesia on an outpatient basis, and rarely will the patient be able to feel anything during the operation itself. Occasionally, after certain procedures (such as refractive surgery) are completed, the patient may experience mild to moderate short-term discomfort. Other modern ophthalmic procedures (such as laser therapy) cause absolutely no pain either during or after surgery because no incisions are made. Recovery time following these new procedures is also quite rapid, with many patients able to resume normal activities almost immediately.

Myth #2: Today's ophthalmic surgery can be used to solve any vision problem, and everyone can benefit from all of the new techniques.

Fact: While ophthalmologists can perform the new high-tech procedures described in this book to help patients with cataracts, glaucoma, certain refractive errors, and many retinal problems, these techniques are not a cureall and they are not for everyone. Some patients' cataracts are simply not suitable for removal by phacoemulsification, for example, and some patients' refractive errors do not fall within the limits that can be corrected by refractive surgery. Most common eye diseases and vision disorders *can* be treated by these new procedures, however, but only an ophthalmologist can make that determination after completing a thorough eye exam.

Myth #3: Eye surgery is most effective when it is performed in a standard hospital setting, where the patient can recuperate for several days before returning home.

Fact: The proliferation and growing use of outpatient surgery centers throughout the United States, particularly for ophthalmic procedures, has shown that surgery no longer must be accompanied by an overnight hospital stay in order to be safe and effective. Despite the fact that in-hospital surgery was the accepted method for all operations until quite recently, a number of nationwide studies have indicated that outpatient surgery can actually be more beneficial to both patient and physician. In addition, most of the ophthalmic procedures in widespread use today generally do not require lengthy recuperation periods.

Myth #4: Postoperative patients will be required to severely restrict their general activities following eye surgery, and they may never be able to resume their preoperative lifestyle.

Fact: Because of their relatively primitive nature, some ophthalmic surgical procedures used in years past often *did* necessitate a lengthy and restricted convalescence. Cataract patients, for example, were instructed to neither tie their shoelaces nor lift heavy objects for fear that the surgeon's work would come undone. However, because of today's microsurgical techniques (which require smaller incisions and thus fewer sutures) and ophthalmic lasers (which require no sutures at all), these restrictions no longer exist. Patients usually return home directly after surgery and most can resume normal activities almost immediately. Eye surgery no longer means an end to the patient's established lifestyle.

Myth #5: All eye surgery patients must wear an eyepatch for long periods of time following their operation.

Fact: Eyepatches are only required after certain procedures—usually those in which an incision is required—and even then they can usually be removed on the day after surgery.

MYTHS ABOUT CATARACTS

Myth #6: Cataracts are a tumor or a film that covers the eye.

Fact: Cataracts are actually a clouding of the eye's normally clear crystalline lens, and an individual is said to develop a cataract when this lens becomes so dark that light rays cannot be transmitted easily through it. Most cataracts occur as a natural part of the aging process, although they also can result from injury, infection, disease, birth defects, or hereditary factors.

Myth #7: Cataracts can go away by themselves.

Fact: Left untreated, over time cataracts will in fact get worse and continually decrease a patient's vision. In the past, many physicians have tried various medical treatments, eye drops, and dietary modifications to prevent or to clear up cataracts, but today it is known that the only way to remove them is through surgery.

Myth #8: Cataracts must be allowed to "ripen" before they can be extracted.

Fact: Before the widespread use of ophthalmic microsurgery, most patients were required to wait until their cataracts "ripened" or matured before successful surgery could even be attempted. Because of today's high-tech methods of extraction, however, this is no longer the case and a cataract can be removed whenever it begins to affect the patient's normal activities. The best time for cataract surgery is now determined by the patient himself in consultation with his ophthalmologist. It is no longer necessary for a patient to wait until he cannot see anything out of his afflicted eye. Many ophthalmologists suggest that cataract surgery should be scheduled whenever the patient finds that his problem is beginning to interfere with regular daily activities.

Myth #9: Cataracts can be removed by a laser.
Fact: The only proven methods for cataract removal are three related processes known as intracapsular extraction, extracapsular extraction, and phacoemulsification, none of which utilizes a laser. However, a neodymium-YAG laser may be used at some point *after* certain extracapsular extractions, because a portion of the lens capsule that has been intentionally left in the eye may develop a clouding or "wrinkling" in approximately one-fifth of all cases. In the past, this problem could only be corrected by additional ophthalmic surgery; today, it can be quickly treated with a laser, often right in the ophthalmologist's office.

Myth #10: An eye can sustain damage if it is used too much after cataract surgery.
Fact: Patients who undergo modern methods of cataract extraction can return almost immediately to the activities and lifestyle that they enjoyed prior to their operation. The postoperative cataract patient cannot damage his eye through use, and no such restrictions are ever required.

Myth #11: After it has been implanted, an intraocular lens may be rejected by the body.
Fact: When they first appeared on the scene, some early intraocular lenses did occasionally cause a problem known as *toxic lens syndrome,* but this has been eliminated through advanced technology and continual improvements. Today's IOLs are composed of inert materials that cannot be rejected by the eye, and it is estimated that they are now safely implanted in from 75 to 90 percent of all cataract patients.

Myth #12: Some patients can obtain "free" cataract surgery.

Fact: In recent years, numerous ophthalmologists around the country have begun advertising that they will perform free or "no cost" cataract surgery for Medicare patients, a claim that leads many skeptics to dismiss these physicians as hucksters who cannot possibly deliver what they promise. Nonetheless, once a patient's yearly Medicare deductible has been met, surgery for cataracts may indeed be performed without additional out-of-pocket costs to the patient. Physicians must individually review all cases in which a patient can demonstrate financial hardship, for example; after such a review, the physician may not require his patient to pay any fees or charges that Medicare has not covered. Cataract surgery is never "free," however, and someone (patient, physician, insurance carrier, or a combination of the three) will be paying the cost.

Myth #13: After cataracts have developed, a patient's eyesight will never again be very good.

Fact: Today's methods of cataract extraction have proven highly successful and more than 95 percent of the patients who undergo them regain useful vision. This restoration of proper sight has been dramatically aided in recent years by the implantation of an intraocular lens, which offers the patient maintenance-free vision restoration with minimal magnification and distortion, good depth perception, and full peripheral vision. Many patients, in fact, find that their postoperative vision is much better than it had been for years prior to surgery.

MYTHS CONCERNING REFRACTIVE ERRORS

Myth #14: Reading in dim light or sitting too close to the TV can damage the eyes.

Fact: Generally, vision problems are either hereditary, caused by some type of injury, or the result of the natural aging process. While prescription lenses for refractive errors like nearsightedness and farsightedness must be updated periodically, this is because the patient's entire body, including the eye, continually changes and matures. There is no evidence that any eye disease or vision disorder is caused by dim reading light or proximity to the television, although these activities certainly can lead to problems such as headaches.

Myth #15: A farsighted person can see distant objects clearly without any corrective lenses.

Fact: Even though the term *farsighted* is the opposite of the term *nearsighted,* the two refractive errors do not necessarily lead to opposite vision problems. Since a farsighted individual has an eyeball that is too short and a retina that is located too far forward, light rays from nearby objects generally will not be properly focused. (Nearsighted people have eyes that are too long and therefore cannot focus light properly from distant objects.) However, many farsighted adults find that their particular problem leaves them unable to see either nearby or distant objects clearly without the use of prescription lenses. Ironically, the flexibility of the crystalline lens in the eyes of farsighted children often can compensate for this deficiency and they can see well at both distances without the need for corrective lenses.

Myth #16: Astigmatic patients cannot be fitted with soft or extended-wear contact lenses.

Fact: Until a few years ago, astigmatic patients were forced to settle for prescription eyeglasses or hard contact lenses; the soft lenses that were available were of no use because they would eventually conform to the cornea's irregularities and merely copy the patient's existing refractive error. However, development of a newer type of soft contact lens, known as a *toric lens,* alleviated these past problems. These lenses are more difficult to fit correctly and they cost more than conventional contact lenses, but when properly utilized they will provide astigmatic patients with excellent vision correction.

Myth #17: Contact lenses can become lost within the eye or move behind the eyeball.

Fact: Because of the eye's structure, there is absolutely no way for a contact lens to move off the cornea and become located anywhere else within the eyeball. A contact lens can, however, move temporarily off the center of the cornea and become lodged on the sclera (white of the eye) or under an eyelid, both nothing more than minor inconveniences that can be easily and quickly reversed.

Myth #18: Extended-wear contact lenses can be left in all eyes for the same length of time.

Fact: Although several manufacturers advertise that their new extended-wear lenses can be worn for as long as four weeks at a time, ophthalmologists often temper this claim with more conservative advice. Many, in fact, suggest that these increasingly popular lenses be worn for only one or two weeks before removal and cleaning. The recommendations vary further according to an individual patient's own comfort and needs, as well as such factors as local climate. (Patients in humid areas will often be able to wear them for longer periods than will those in dry parts of the country.)

Myth #19: The eye can become so dependent upon contact lenses that the patient will never be able to wear eyeglasses again.

Fact: Contact lenses are convenient, they often provide superior vision correction, and they may dramatically improve a patient's own self-image. However, since the use of contact lenses will neither improve nor worsen a patient's vision, the only dependence that can possibly develop will be a psychological one. Many patients do, in fact, switch regularly between their eyeglasses and their contacts.

Myth #20: The use of prescribed eyeglasses or contact lenses will reverse the effects of a refractive error or keep it from progressing further.

Fact: No reputable scientific evidence has yet been developed to show that corrective lenses can eliminate an existing refractive error, or keep one from worsening over time. A patient's nearsightedness or farsightedness, determined by heredity, will change naturally over the years as the body matures and ages. Nothing except one of the new refractive surgical procedures can alter this fact.

MYTHS ABOUT OTHER EYE DISORDERS

Myth #21: Damage to the optic nerve that results from glaucoma can be surgically reversed.

Fact: Glaucoma remains one of the leading causes of blindness in the United States precisely because such damage, once it occurs, *cannot* be reversed. Only prompt diagnosis and treatment can prevent a loss of vision due to this disease, which strikes about two percent of those over age forty.

Myth #22: Detached retinas are generally suffered only by boxers and other athletes who are involved in rugged contact sports.

Fact: This sight-threatening problem, which develops when the retina separates from its adjoining layer, can result from several distinct causes. A blow to the eye, as experienced by participants in certain rough physical activities, is only one of them—although, because of the public nature of such a sports-related injury, it may receive the greatest share of attention. Other possible factors include a cyst or tumor in the eye, scar tissue, a hemorrhage, an infection or other eye disease, and the inescapable fact that an aging eye's vitreous humor may adhere to the retina and then begin shrinking. The problem is actually most common in those over age fifty who suffer from nearsightedness.

Myth #23: Detached retinas can be repaired with the aid of a laser.

Fact: If the retinal holes or tears that precede a complete detachment are detected in time, an eye surgeon can aim an argon laser directly through the patient's pupil and create an adhesive scar that will coagulate the separating layers. If a detachment has already occurred, the use of other ophthalmic surgical procedures may be necessary.

MYTHS ABOUT BASIC EYE CARE

Myth #24: Good nutrition or specialized diets alone can prevent eye disease.

Fact: Eye diseases usually result from factors beyond the control of the patient. Likewise, these diseases usually cannot be stopped or prevented without ophthalmic intervention. Although in the past some special diets have been tried for patients with problems such as cataracts and retinopathy, no successful efforts have been recorded. The mistaken belief stretches back to the time when it was honestly thought that carrots could be eaten to improve vision because they are rich in Vitamin A, an ingredient essential for sight. However, only a small amount of Vitamin A is necessary for good vision, and that is usually supplied by a well-balanced diet. Nonetheless, various dietary modifications to improve eyesight will probably be the subject of new experimental efforts in years to come.

Myth #25: The regular use of eye exercises will improve poor eyesight and eliminate existing vision disorders.

Fact: Just as some people mistakenly believe that dietary habits can influence the development and progression of eye disease, others incorrectly assume that various exercises can prove useful in the battle against vision disorders. Over the years, in fact, articles and even entire books have appeared to proclaim that premise. Despite our optimism, however, not one of these efforts has been successfully supported by scientific research. The only proven way to treat existing eye ailments is through the use of medication, surgery, or a combination of the two, and the only proven way to improve poor vision is through the use of prescription lenses or refractive surgery.

Myth #26: Eyes can be transplanted.

Fact: At present, the transplantation of an entire eye is not possible. Visual images are transmitted from the eye to the brain by way of the optic nerve, and if this delicate link is severed it cannot be reconnected. However, efforts to transplant the cornea have proven successful, leading some people to believe that the entire eye can be replaced.

Myth #27: Sitting all day before a video display terminal (VDT) will lead to vision damage, possible internal injuries, or both.

Fact: No evidence has yet been uncovered to prove that prolonged computer usage will damage the eyes or result in other physical injuries. However, because of the manner in which they are used, many of those who work with a computer for long, uninterrupted periods routinely complain of eyestrain, headaches, and other general ailments. Usually, these conditions can be alleviated by regular breaks. If symptoms persist, an examination by an ophthalmologist is in order.

8

The Outpatient Surgery Boom

Until a few years ago, nearly all surgical procedures were governed by a rigid set of rules. The most prominent feature among these rules was a staunch requirement that all surgical patients, with very few exceptions, were to be hospitalized automatically for several days or even longer at the time their operation was scheduled. This strict routine may have raised an occasional eyebrow here and there, but the few doctors and patients who questioned the need for hospitalization were rarely effective at having their objections and concerns recognized.

Under these standard operating procedures, the patient was first directed to a hospital that was most often selected by his physician. He would be admitted to this hospital on one day for an operation that would generally be performed on the next. Depending on the complexity of the surgery and the seriousness of his condition, the patient would then be allowed to return to his home anytime from the third to the seventh day following his initial admittance.

With a few notable exceptions, this procedure had become accepted over the years for practically every type of surgery from cataract extraction to gallstone removal. Patients, who often had friends and relatives that shared a similar experience, saw no reason to question it. Surgeons, who required access to these hospitals' state-of-the-art operating equipment, really could not afford to complain. Hospitals, which make their money depending upon how many beds they fill, obviously could find nothing wrong with the system. Even the insurance companies, which pay the vast majority of surgical bills, did not argue with something that was so strongly supported by everyone else.

But, during the last decade, a few significant changes took place that suddenly and dramatically altered this long-standard practice. All at once, it seemed, the old set of rules was being rewritten and automatic overnight hospitalization for many procedures was no longer routinely prescribed. There was some initial and anticipated opposition to the change, of course, but most of those involved now believe that the transformation that resulted was a good thing from every point of view.

THE RULES WERE REWRITTEN

It's not surprising that the astounding amount of money spent on medical care in recent years was the primary reason that the old rules were finally rewritten. When America's per capita spending on health care reached $2,580 in the mid-1980s, up three times from 1974 levels, the situation had become worse than alarming. Automatic overnight hospitalization was identified as one of the main reasons for a downward slide in the profits of many private insurance companies, as well as for much of the financial entanglement experienced by the federal government's Medicare program, which is the largest provider of health-care benefits in the nation. With so much at stake, a few insurers decided to study the problem and then take action.

Watching their payouts soar as medical costs continued to

skyrocket, these insurers wondered whether certain relatively common procedures really necessitated a week-long stay in a high-priced hospital room. After talking to scores of physicians and patients, they determined that many operations actually did *not* require hospitalization, even for one night. Led by Medicare, a number of prominent insurance providers then began to discourage the long-time practice of automatic overnight hospitalization by refusing to routinely pay for it, unless it could be shown that a hospital stay was really required for the patient's health.

At about the same time, certain innovative surgeons also started to question the system in which they had become involuntary participants. Some had long questioned the value of automatically hospitalizing their patients for various routine procedures, but they followed the old rules because there was nowhere else to perform the surgery. Others had long questioned the necessity of always performing these procedures in a high-priced hospital setting, but they, too, followed the crowd because they needed the hospital's facilities in order to operate.

Then, two things happened that helped to provide a solid answer for many of those surgeons who were questioning the long hospital stays. The first came when insurers began to discourage automatic hospitalization. The second and, for the surgeons, more significant event came when space-age tools like lasers and operating microscopes arrived on the scene at affordable prices. Physicians who had been seeking an alternative knew it had arrived. Some built outpatient operating facilities right in their own offices, while others joined with colleagues to create large, private ambulatory surgery centers.

With these two major forces now actively teaming up against the old system, a number of hospitals themselves realized they had to get into the act—and quickly. Not wanting to alienate either insurers or surgeons, these hospitals worked to develop their own alternatives for a variety of low-risk procedures that would help to keep their facilities operating but eliminate the need for automatic overnight hospitalizations. They created their own outpatient centers, sometimes right within the hospital and other times in freestanding buildings. To-day, more than 70 percent of all hospitals in the United States have outpatient centers of their own, and insurers estimate that these and similar private facilities eventually will cut the cost of health care by as much as 50 percent.

Medical Costs Had Been Ignored

Considering today's high-priced medical care, this significant cost-saving factor should not be underestimated. Un-til just a few years ago, the prevailing American attitude about medicine generally held that good care is expensive and better care is more expensive. Coupled with an unfortunate trend that resulted in a number of insurance plans that often covered 100 percent of a patient's medical bills even when this total coverage was not warranted, the incentive to shop for high-quality, low-cost medical care was all but lost.

While this lack of consumer awareness would have been rejected in almost any other area of American life, in medicine it was somehow condoned. Patients armed with an ill-conceived attitude and a full-coverage medical plan sought care with absolutely no regard toward its cost. Top care was critical, they reasoned, and expense was irrelevant.

Rather than being seen as the unneccessary expense that it often was, therefore, automatic overnight hospitalization was simply viewed as another one of the great benefits to which the patient was entitled. But even as many of us wrongly con-sidered these and other benefits that were covered by our in-surance plans to be "free," we were actually paying for them all along. Now that the problem has boosted health-care costs to the point where they consume more than 12 percent of the United States' Gross National Product, the cry for cost reduction has become loud. And the switch from inpatient to outpatient surgery has been one important response.

Despite the clear economic benefits that outpatient sur-gery seems to offer, however, this change never would be sup-ported unless it also offered a clear continuation of our existing tradition of excellence in medical care. Fortunately for all of us, it already has been proven that the push toward outpatient surgery will *not* lead to a sacrifice in the quality of care we have come to expect. As the use of outpatient surgery centers has become widespread during the last several years, in fact, a variety of nationwide studies repeatedly has shown them to be beneficial for both patient and surgeon.

Patients and Physicians Are Enthusiastic

Patients who have utilized them are their greatest advocates. Since most of us do not enjoy going to a hospital even when the trip may be absolutely necessary, it also should not surprise us to learn that patients are enthusiastic about a system that permits them to return home as little as two hours after arriving for surgery. Recent surveys indicate that when given the choice today, most of us now prefer outpatient surgery as long as we can be assured of getting the same quality of care and excellence in results that we anticipate receiving in a hospital setting. In fact, only those without any outpatient experience at all, either personally or through a friend or family member, still feel that they are unsatisfactory alternatives.

Physicians, too, have shown a marked preference for the new outpatient settings. Since these surgical facilities generally have been built only within the last few years, the equipment that is installed there is as modern and up-to-date as that found anywhere else. Therefore, the surgeons still have access to the latest in lasers, diagnostic computers, and high-tech examination instruments, a fact which has helped to negate many of the arguments initially advanced when the trend against automatic overnight hospitalization first began.

Also, many physicians have been pleased to discover that in an outpatient center they now have more control over the total environment in which they operate. They can, for example, provide input on everything from the hiring of a nursing staff to the purchase of sutures. While this new attention to every single detail admittedly does add to the huge burden of responsibility already present upon the surgeon's shoulders, it also places the control of all relevant factors in the hands of those who ultimately are responsible for them, but who often had little direct say about them in the past.

EYE SURGERY IS THE BENEFICIARY

With all of these advantages it really is little wonder that outpatient surgery has caught on so strongly—especially in the field of ophthalmology, which is perhaps more of a technology-oriented specialty than any other branch of medicine. Most eye surgery procedures, after all, are quite simple and safe when they are performed under the direction of a qualified ophthalmologist. Even though most of these procedures required an automatic overnight hospitalization as recently as a few years ago, the advent of advanced ophthalmic tools and techniques has allowed outpatient surgery to take a firm hold.

The evidence of the shift to outpatient surgery in today's ophthalmology is striking, particularly in the area of cataract extraction. It is estimated, for example, that fewer than ten percent of all cataract surgeries now being performed in the United States are still done in an inpatient hospital setting. A late 1985 survey of some 4,500 ophthalmologists who routinely implant an intraocular lens in their patient's eye following cataract extraction indicated that nearly 72 percent performed their surgery in a hospital outpatient clinic, almost 14 percent operated in an ambulatory surgery center, and just over 4 percent extracted the cataract right in their own office.

THREE TYPES OF FACILITIES

As the system has developed over the past few years, there are now basically three different places where outpatient surgery can be performed: the hospital-based outpatient facility, the ambulatory surgery center, and the physician's office itself. While each one of these is different from the others and tends to offer its own set of advantages, they all contrast significantly with the old inpatient system in which the patient was admitted to a hospital room where he had to remain for several days. Despite their variations, under all three of these outpatient alternatives the patient can expect to undergo surgery shortly after his arrival and then be released for home shortly after his operation.

Perhaps because of their direct and obvious relationship with the traditional medical system to which most of us have become accustomed over the years, many patients find that they are most comfortable with a hospital-based outpatient facility. To many of us, after all, the operations that are performed under these conditions will seem almost identical to the inpatient system that was common in years past.

Today's increasing trend toward private outpatient centers has intensified the competition between those who provide health care in America. While good location and modern equipment still may be an important part of a hospital's total package, these benefits certainly can be equaled or even bettered by many of the private centers that are springing up around the country. If a patient chooses a hospital-based outpatient facility for his surgery, therefore, it should be selected because that center will provide him with the best care that is available, and not simply because it is part of a hospital.

The Biggest Change

Perhaps the biggest change to come about as a result of this trend toward outpatient treatment is the development and popularity of an entirely new kind of facility known as the *ambulatory surgery center.* While these freestanding clinics—named as they are because they treat nonbedridden patients who are able to walk in and walk out—often look just like a hospital on the inside, they generally tend to be much smaller in scale and therefore more efficient and more comfortable from the patient's point of view. A carefully planned and staffed outpatient center of this kind, however, also will provide medical treatment that is as safe and as effective as that offered in any other type of facility.

Although in recent years, an ambulatory surgery center has come to mean different things to different people—or even very little to those of us who still are unfamiliar with the relatively new concept—the term really does represent a wide variety of out-patient choices. These centers can be owned and operated by a hospital, for example, or they can be run by a lone surgeon or a group of physicians who have banded together for this particular venture. They can handle patients seeking care from a number of different medical specialties, or they can concentrate exclusively on only one specific field like ophthalmology or orthopedics. They can be part of a group of such centers, or the only one of their kind.

One of the nation's first ambulatory surgery centers was constructed in 1969 in Phoenix, Arizona. Today, over 250 of these efficient and ultramodern facilities are located in practically every part of the United States. As the knowledge of their benefits continues to spread among both patients and physicians, more and more are being planned every day.

HOW TO CHOOSE

Patients who are interested in this type of facility and are seeking the highest quality of care that is available can check first for the existence of a specific center's state or federal licensing. Although the actual regulations for operating a surgical center of this nature can vary greatly from state to state, these centers must pass a number of national or local requirements in order to qualify for reimbursement by Medicare and most private insurance companies. Since few can afford to operate without these reimbursements, most reputable centers will routinely seek such licensing before they open.

Struggling through the maze of confusing and often-contradictory rules and regulations can be another matter, however, for both the operators of these centers and those who wish to utilize their services. Only about half of all fifty states currently have their own requirements for licensing, for example, while the others rely solely on federal regulations. This could mean that while plans for a center may be sufficient to earn it a license in one state, the identical proposal may not enable a center's operators to obtain a license in an adjoining state. Still, possession of state or federal licenses does indicate that the center in question has complied with a variety of strict standards and qualifications and most likely will provide high-quality care.

There are numerous advantages to be gained by choosing to undergo an operation in an ambulatory surgery center. First, because the vast majority of these centers have been built in only the last few years, they often contain only the latest, most modern equipment. Second, because they are designed to compete with hospitals and other existing health-care delivery systems, they usually are constructed in only the most convenient locations. Third, because they are relatively small-scale operations, they generally are free from the red tape and bureaucracy that can be the downfall of many larger institutions.

Perhaps the most important advantage, however, concerns their exclusive practice of outpatient surgery in only one or a small number of procedures. While a hospital operating room may see a dozen patients admitted for a dozen different operations on any one given day, an ambulatory surgery center may see only a dozen cataract patients or a dozen refractive surgery patients on that same day. Because of this specialization, therefore, ambulatory surgery centers and their staffs tend to become very good at what they do.

The third and final type of outpatient facility that is available to patients today is located right in the doctor's office. Because of the advanced tools and techniques that now highlight many specialties, including ophthalmology, some procedures can be performed by the physician and his assistant in the same room that usually is used for examinations and other forms of treatment. While a number of complicated procedures cannot be done in this type of setting, certain operations (like ophthalmic laser surgery) can be performed quickly and easily under these more informal conditions.

Since no one looks forward to any type of operation, the primary advantage to undergoing surgery in a physician's office is the familiar setting and familiar staff. Here, the patient can enter a facility in which he already feels comfortable. He can deal with a surgeon and support staff he already has learned to trust. And since the office most likely is located near the patient's home, he can make the trip to and from the operation without the possible anxiety that could accompany his traveling to some faraway and unfamiliar facility.

SOME OBSTACLES STILL EXIST

While the growing national trend toward outpatient surgery has proven beneficial in almost every location to which it has spread, certain states have not made it easy for centers that wish to do business within their borders. State laws regarding these facilities vary greatly and not all local governments have proven receptive to outpatient centers that are not owned by hospitals. An inability to obtain needed certification in these states has presented a continual problem for both proposed centers and the patients who could benefit from their existence.

Most observers attribute the problem to numerous powerful, local hospital lobbies. They recognize that almost all hospitals are suffering from their own financial problems these days, and few of these institutions therefore welcome the prospect of added competition. Since hospitals generally are regarded as highly respected businesses in the communities in which they function, offering a stable supply of good jobs in addition to much-needed medical care, their concerns about competition usually are met by receptive ears.

Continued pressure from physicians, patients, and insurance companies is beginning to change this, however, as leading spokesmen for all three groups now fully accept the high quality of care and the cost savings that can be found through proper outpatient care. Eventually, it is believed, the resistance that still exists in several states will be squashed and private outpatient centers will be permitted to take up residence there. But then, and only then, will citizens in all parts of the United States be free to benefit from what may be the greatest change in medical care to occur this century—outpatient surgery.

Outpatient centers themselves, of course, are responsible for upholding the high standards of medical care that today's patients have come to expect. Every task they perform, from surgery to record keeping to house cleaning, must be equal to or better than that found in traditional hospitals. After convincing patients that quality care need not be expensive, outpatient centers must also prove that cost saving need not mean sacrifice.

Over time, more and more of these clinics will be constructed across the country and outpatient surgery will grow in acceptance. As this happens, the opportunity for unscrupulous operators to enter the picture will also grow. Fair but firm regulations should keep all but qualified centers from opening, however, and the increase in competition will intensify the pressure to provide an unwavering level of excellent care. Like other businesses, centers that are able to meet these high standards will survive and prosper.

HOW OUTPATIENT FACILITIES WORK

In most centers where outpatient surgery is performed, the day of surgery itself is marked by a fairly predictable pattern that varies only slightly from standard inpatient proceedings. Usually, the patient already has been briefed on his operation during an earlier visit, at which time he also was given a specific arrival time for surgery, just as if he were scheduled for an inpatient operation. One major difference, however, is that he will not be required to bring any clothes or personal items along because he will be returning home shortly after the operation. Another difference is that, especially with certain ophthalmic procedures, he may be advised to bring a friend or relative along who can drive him home after surgery.

Once the patient and his companion have arrived at the appointed hour and been greeted by the center's staff, the patient will usually be taken into the facility's prep room in order to be prepared for surgery. Here, he will be asked to change out of his streetclothes and his vital signs will be checked; often, he also will be rebriefed on the procedure that is about to take place. Additionally, if it is necessary for this operation, the staff may now begin to administer topical anesthesia as well as eye drops to dilate the patient's pupils.

When the actual time for surgery arrives, the patient will be taken into an operating room that looks exactly like the most up-to-date inpatient facility that would be found today in the finest of hospitals. After reclining on an operating table, the patient will be covered by a surgical drape while his physician and several support personnel take up their positions around him. An operating microscope will be moved into place, and the surgery will begin, usually with the patient completely awake and conscious of his surroundings.

Although a specific procedure itself will vary little from outpatient center to outpatient center, a small but growing number of facilities will provide the friend or relative who is awaiting its conclusion with a unique and definitely high-tech option. These centers have equipped their operating suites with a video camera that is linked to a viewing screen, at which the patient's companion can sit and watch the entire operation if he so chooses. A few of these monitored centers will even present their patients with a videotape of the entire procedure that they can take home as a memento of their visit! As unusual as this may sound, physicians report that some patients actually do request a copy of this offbeat home movie.

Once the surgery has been completed—and many ophthalmic procedures take only twenty or thirty minutes—the patient is taken to a recovery area where he will be reunited with his companion and offered something to eat and drink. After a specified resting period and instructions on postoperative care, he will be permitted to leave for home. Usually, the entire period of time that has elapsed from his initial arrival to his eventual departure will run no longer than two hours.

THE OUTPATIENT EYE SURGERY BOOM

Perhaps the most common ophthalmic procedure now performed regularly under outpatient conditions is the cataract removal, 90 percent of which are undertaken today in outpatient facilities of one kind or another. Especially in the hands of modern eye surgeons who favor extracapsular cataract extraction or the more technically demanding phacoemulsification method, these relatively rapid outpatient procedures have proven to be extremely safe and successful. They also offer a negligible complication rate and their accompanying physical discomfort is much less than that associated with other forms of surgery.

The laser surgery that is sometimes necessary after the completion of these forms of cataract extraction, required when the remaining posterior lens capsule clouds up or wrinkles, also is a made-to-order outpatient procedure. Since this development occurs in about 20 percent of all patients, before the advent of ophthalmic lasers it tended to curtail the use of extracapsular extraction and phacoemulsification. But a few painless bursts from the powerful neodymium-YAG laser, without the need for an invasive surgical incision, can now clear up this common problem in a matter of moments.

Without a doubt, lasers have been a primary reason for the proliferation and success of outpatient eye surgery. While glaucoma remains one of the leading causes of blindness in the United States, for example, several new high-tech surgical treatments involving the argon laser have proven very effective in curtailing its potential damage. When the disease is caught in time and drug therapy does not seem to work, two painless outpatient laser procedures have been used successfully to halt glaucoma's otherwise inevitable destruction of the eye's optic nerve.

A variety of potentially sight-threatening retinal problems are also being treated regularly now by means of outpatient laser therapy. A trio of these ailments—macular degeneration, retinal tears, and diabetic retinopathy—all have responded particularly well to the argon or krypton laser. Continuing developments in this area also promise that even more effective outpatient treatments for retinal disorders may be available in the near future.

Not all of the ophthalmic procedures that are effective in outpatient settings involve lasers, however. A number of the most promising and exciting now are being used to surgically correct the eye's three main refractive errors by "remodeling" the patient's cornea. Despite the remarkable nature of these space-age procedures, they, too, usually are performed on an outpatient basis.

WHY GO TO A HOSPITAL?

With all of the significant medical and sociological advantages that have been associated with outpatient surgery, many people must wonder why all operations are not performed on that basis today. The response to that question is not as complicated as it may initially seem, although the reasons behind the answer certainly are complex.

First of all, proper outpatient facilities still are not available in all areas of the country. In some places, this is caused by numerous regulatory entanglements that occasionally prove insurmountable. No one is suggesting that regulations are a bad idea; sometimes, in fact, strict rules have even been proposed by advocates of outpatient surgery. The problem instead lies with the absence of clear and unbiased outpatient regulations in certain parts of the nation that effectively keeps such facilities from being built in those areas. Ironically, other communities lack an appropriate center simply because no one has gotten around to building one yet. And then there are areas where excellent outpatient centers already exist, but which may not be technically capable—or adequately staffed—to perform every single type of surgical procedure.

Secondly, a number of common and not-so-common surgical procedures still are considered to be safest and most effective when they are performed in an inpatient hospital setting. Some operations, for example, absolutely require a postoperative recovery period that can be monitored continuously by a trained hospital staff. Other operative procedures still have not advanced, either technically or technologically, to the point where they can be performed regularly on an outpatient basis. As additional improvements are made in coming years, however, the number and variety of procedures that can be performed in outpatient clinics is expected to expand significantly.

Finally, outpatient surgery simply is not right for every patient, regardless of the procedure that is scheduled and the facilities that are available. Those who suffer from serious problems like a heart condition, for example, always should be operated upon in a fully equipped hospital in the event that something goes wrong during surgery. Other patients whose general health is less than perfect—including those with high blood pressure, diabetes, or a tendency towards bleeding—also may find an inpatient procedure to be less risky. Additionally, patients who do not have someone at home to help them recover after an outpatient operation may find their convalescence more effective under the supervision of a hospital staff.

IS OUTPATIENT SURGERY THE ANSWER?

In most situations, the patient's physician will be the one to initially recommend or reject an outpatient procedure. Unfortunately, however, not every physician is knowledgable about the latest in outpatient care. In these cases, it falls upon the patient's shoulders to discover the variety of procedures that can be performed in this manner, as well as the outpatient facilities that are available within the nearby community. If the physician still will not provide the information and guidance that is sought by his patient, it probably is time to seek a new physician or at least a second opinion.

This new ability to actively participate in our own medical future is important to all of us. No longer are we as patients tied down to the rigid rules of order that have governed medicine for hundreds of years. Today, those of us who are informed about our conditions and our alternatives can make a significant impact on the type of care we are to receive. This goes for simple office evaluations as well as surgery. The old set of regulations—including those dreaded and unneccessary automatic overnight hospitalizations for nearly every type of surgical procedure—have been banished, thankfully, forever.

Many of these changes have come about as a direct result of the spread of outpatient surgery, which has been acknowledged as one of the most signiciant medical advances of our time. As this practice slowly but steadily moves into every corner of our society, the field of ophthalmology will continue to help lead the way. With these and other medical improvements coming as quickly and significantly as they are today, it is difficult to predict what the future may hold. However, in the next chapter, we offer an educated guess.

9

Eye Surgery Of The Future

If we could transport a pre–World War II eye surgeon into the 1980s, we would graphically see just how much this specialty has evolved during the last few decades. For after simply examining the current state of his branch of medicine, our time-traveling ophthalmologist would probably go into shock.

During his time, after all, there was no such thing as an operating microscope or microsurgery. Cataracts, glaucoma, and retinal disorders were treated with a variety of primitive procedures that often proved unsuccessful. Refractive errors were corrected exclusively with prescription eyeglasses. Lasers were as far-fetched as space travel. And surgery outside a hospital was absolutely unthinkable.

Few prewar physicians could have envisioned the radical changes that have taken place in ophthalmology, and today's eye surgeons are equally at a loss to predict the state of their specialty some forty years hence. All indications, however, lead observers to believe that the next few decades will bring about even more earth-shaking developments than the ones that have occurred in the recent past.

Today's ophthalmology has been shaped by its vastly improved instruments and procedures, and tomorrow's ophthalmology will be marked by a number of similar developments. Tools and techniques introduced during the last few decades are continually being refined and updated, and amazing advances once considered only hopeful dreams are now nearing reality. But because these improvements are occurring at such a rapid rate, an educated guess as to what the future might hold is just that—an educated guess. Nonetheless, an examination of the current trends in ophthalmic experimentation can help us to understand the direction that this still-evolving future may ultimately take.

EXPERIMENTATION GOES ON

A vast array of experimental tools and techniques that ultimately might improve the exciting procedures now being used in eye surgery are under continual evaluation, and some of the most beneficial eventually may prove safe and successful and thus gain approval for general use. This ongoing experimentation is taking place all over the world, with results presented at ophthalmology meetings or reported periodically in ophthalmology journals.

These studies—which are often very preliminary—are scrutinized carefully and commented upon extensively by the researcher's peers, some of whom may be working simultaneously on similar projects. This lengthy process of experimentation and evaluation then continues until the new project either is embraced as satisfactory or abandoned as unsuccessful. Only when other members of the ophthalmic community are satisfied with the results, however, are any of these new tools or techniques made available to the public.

The preliminary experiments on proposed new instruments and procedures frequently are conducted on animals, even though few animals make perfect subjects. A rabbit's eye, for example, contains a proportionately larger lens than a human's, and it is able to reproduce endothelial cells of the cornea while a human eye cannot. But since it is not completely safe to perform early ophthalmic experimentation directly on human eyes, researchers are forced to utilize the closest model that they can obtain.

Once this initial animal research indicates that a new tool or a new technique may indeed have some merit, its prospects for acceptance are increased. At that time, it becomes necessary to test the new instrument or procedure on a variety of carefully chosen human volunteers. These tests are called *clinical trials* and are conducted according to a strict scientific method so that the results can be accurately measured, studied, and compared. If these results also prove unquestionably positive, this new option soon may be adopted by some eye surgeons.

The purpose of this painstakingly careful review process is to ensure that only the safest and most promising of all the new developments eventually are utilized by ophthalmologists around the country. For this reason, patients can assume that even though a particular procedure may be criticized by certain physicians, if it is being performed on the public, it has received the approval of a large segment of the general ophthalmic community.

TWO AREAS OFFER GREATEST HOPE

Since much of today's experimentation deals with proposed advances in surgery for cataracts and refractive errors, these studies offer the most hope for the greatest number of tomorrow's patients. In fact, many of the millions who will seek help for these disorders in the future actually may be offered a variety of new treatment alternatives that are light-years ahead of today's very successful high-tech options.

A large percentage of today's ongoing studies are concerned with proposed improvements to intraocular lenses and ophthalmic lasers, with some researchers attempting to create completely new technology while others try to develop new uses for existing equipment. Although it would not be feasible to describe each and every one of the exciting experiments that are announced or evaluated almost daily, it is nonetheless possible to get an idea of the direction of current research efforts by examining the work that is being performed on several representative tools and techniques.

IOLs Make Big News

For the millions of those who suffer from cataracts, the biggest news on the horizon may be the continuing improvements that researchers are studying in the area of intraocular lens implants (IOLs). Although these tiny plastic lenses have been around for only two decades and in widespread use for just over ten years, the quarter-inch marvels already have revolutionized the way that cataract surgery is performed by surgeons and perceived by patients. As difficult as it may be to believe, however, developments now under study may offer even more significant changes in the near future.

IOLs usually are implanted in the eye near the conclusion of most modern cataract operations, although they actually can be inserted at any time following an extraction. These clear plastic lenses then replace the eye's natural crystalline lens—which, of course, has been removed during surgery—and they help the cornea to focus the incoming light rays that must land properly on the retina in order for clear vision to result. Because these IOLs often are more optically accurate than the natural lens that was removed, many cataract patients find that their postoperative distance vision has been improved dramatically.

Despite the numerous advantages that are associated with today's intraocular lenses, however, some patients are troubled by a significant drawback that currently is linked to all such implants. No matter how successful these IOLs can be in the restoration of distance vision, the patients soon discover that existing lenses are unable to solve the problem of diminished closeup vision that commonly is experienced by those in the prime cataract age group. Even after receiving an implant, therefore, many patients still require a pair of reading glasses in order to counter the inevitable effects of aging on the eye.

Thanks to current research efforts, though, this well-known inconvenience someday may be little more than a historical footnote. One of the most significant recent experiments in proposed intraocular lens technology involves the development and evaluation of a workable implant that has been dubbed the *bifocal IOL*. If these revolutionary new lenses eventually prove to be safe and effective, they would become the first implants able to provide postoperative cataract patients with properly corrected closeup and distant vision simultaneously.

Although their concept is based on an existing design that currently is used for bifocal contact lenses, the actual production of these advanced IOLs only became feasible when significant improvements were made in the lens manufacturing process. If ongoing studies now show them to be as safe and effective as the lenses already in use, these bifocal IOLs soon may make reading glasses a thing of the past for the vast number of patients who now opt for an intraocular lens implant at the time of cataract surgery.

IOLs For Children

Another of the most exciting areas of current IOL experimentation concerns the ongoing study of investigational silicone implants that eventually may prove feasible for use in children. This news is particularly significant to the scores of young patients who could benefit greatly from a so-called *pediatric implantation,* which generally has been discouraged by most ophthalmologists since the introduction of IOLs.

The reason that most eye surgeons have been reluctant to utilize IOLs among younger patients basically is two-fold, and results mostly from their initial experiences with the technology when it was relatively new. Their fears stem partly from an unacceptable complication rate that is associated with the earliest intraocular lenses, and partly from the fact that for many years, no long-term research was available to show how a young eye will react to implants over a period of five or six decades.

Experimental pediatric implants with a variety of different IOLs has continued over the years, however, because children who are in need of artificial lenses often have a great deal of difficulty with the only other alternative—contact lenses. If evaluations of the current studies involving silicon lenses show that they will provide good visual improvement with few complications, a number of vision-impaired children soon may be able to benefit from the amazing IOL technology that already has enabled millions of older cataract patients to regain excellent eyesight.

Refractive Surgery Marches On

For the countless Americans who suffer from the three major refractive errors, the biggest news in experimental ophthalmology may be the continuing advances that researchers are constantly announcing in refractive surgical tools and techniques. Although it has only been about a decade since eye surgeons first began regularly performing refractive procedures in this country, the acceptance and demand for these new techniques has been so great that ophthalmologists are consistently pressed to develop new and better instruments and methods.

Today, the most commonly performed refractive surgeries in the United States are radial keratotomy (RK), myopic keratomeleusis (MKM), and hyperopic keratomeleusis (HKM). All three are proven, high-tech procedures in which the operating ophthalmologist actually reshapes his patient's cornea in an attempt to correct an existing defect in its curvature. Currently, RKs are performed with the aid of a diamond knife; MKMs and HKMs are performed with a cryolathe. In all cases, the corneal reshaping is guided by computer.

On the investigational front, the *excimer laser* from Germany shows great promise for those moderately nearsighted patients who hope to someday free themselves from eyeglasses or contact lenses by undergoing a radial keratotomy. Preliminary animal studies indicate that the excimer laser safely produces RK incisions that are comparable to those produced by a diamond knife, and may in fact offer several advantages over the existing surgical method.

The excimer laser—whose name is short for "excited dimer"—is a high-powered, short-pulsed source of ultraviolet radiation that combines a gas (such as argon) with a halogen (such as fluorine). Like most other ophthalmic lasers, the excimer is operated by "exciting" this compound (whose union is referred to as a *dimer*) with an electrical discharge in the laser's cavity. Unlike most others, however, the excimer's wavelength can be altered by changing the combination of gas and halogen. Initial research has uncovered a specific wavelength that appears to be the most useful for creating the type of incision that is necessary to perform RKs.

In the hands of a trained eye surgeon, the excimer laser will produce a very thin corneal incision that looks quite similar to the incisions that are produced by a diamond knife. However, current research indicates that the excimer may offer a number of important advantages. These include the ability to cut without making contact and a greatly improved depth control, as well as the fact that the eye surgeon will not have to cut as deeply nor make as many incisions. Potential drawbacks still under study include possible healing problems and the potential for endothelial damage.

Researchers believe that if all of the difficulties can be overcome, including the development of a workable delivery system, the excimer laser will offer both ophthalmologists and their patients the most accurate and efficient RK procedure yet devised. They envision a time when nearsighted patients could be seated before a slit lamp while their preoperative vision data is fed into a computer. Next, all of the necessary incisions would be performed simultaneously by an excimer laser that is attached to the slit lamp until the computer informs the eye surgeon that the desired effect has been achieved. The surgeon then would shut the machine down and the patient would go home.

Other Refractive Techniques Studied

As incredible as that sounds, it also might be possible in the future for certain farsighted individuals to profit from a new technique called *hexagonal keratotomy* that is similar to RK. This investigational procedure is being performed with a diamond knife that places a series of six interconnecting incisions around the optical axis of the cornea in the shape of a hexagon, although it is conceivable that it may also be performed someday with an excimer laser. If this new technique eventually is determined to be safe and effective, it may provide farsighted patients with an additional alternative to corrective lenses and hyperopic keratomeleusis.

Those farsighted patients who do choose to undergo an HKM, however, also may benefit eventually from a series of experiments that are now being evaluated in the United States and West Germany. Currently, eye surgeons who are performing an HKM must remove a section of the patient's cornea, freeze it in a cryolathe, reshape it, and then reattach it. But researchers are studying a new way to perform this operation without freezing the removed corneal section, which would allow it to remain "alive" and thus promote quicker healing. Early experiments indicate that this new alternative may lead to far faster postoperative vision improvement than is possible under the existing technique.

Still another experimental procedure that currently is under investigation may help to improve the vision of a large number of patients who suffer from any of the refractive errors. Using a device that electronically combines an automatic refractometer-keratometer with an excimer-type laser, researchers have found that they can reshape the corneas of those with nearly any degree of nearsightedness, farsightedness, or astigmatism.

Although the instrument still is in very preliminary stages of development, proponents claim that its completely adjustable nature will permit its successful use on a variety of patients who suffer from a wide range of any of these common defects. In addition, they say that its extremely high rate of precision can help eye surgeons to eliminate any of the drawbacks that have become associated with the standard RK, MKM, and HKM procedures.

LASERS WILL SET PACE

Without question, continual advances in laser technology will be setting the pace for the future of ophthalmic surgery. While the most promising of the new procedures may be those performed with the aid of the excimer laser, a number of other promising laser experiments are also being conducted. One involves the dye laser, already proven useful in treating diabetic retinopathy, which may someday be used to treat a variety of retinal problems with a high degree of accuracy. A second, dubbed *fluorescein-antibody laser asepsis,* is a complicated technique that may permit eye surgeons using an argon laser beam to kill all organisms that affect the cornea.

Still another promising new laser technique is one that may prove useful in the future for further improving many cataract extractions. This investigational procedure involves two related techniques—phacofragmentation and phacoemulsification—and is known by the difficult-to-pronounce name of *photophacofragmentation.* It allows the eye surgeon to easily create a small incision that first permits the removal of the contents between the eye's anterior and posterior capsule, and then permits the insertion of a small foldable lens if it is so desired.

APPROVAL BASED ON SAFETY AND EFFECTIVENESS

If any of the exciting new instruments or procedures that are described above—or any of the countless others that are now under evaluation—prove through animal studies and clinical trials to be both safe and effective, they will eventually be approved for general use. And as the public demand for more and better options in high-tech eye surgery continually increases, these new tools and techniques will be improved even further by the many ophthalmologists who are trying to bring additional alternatives to the millions who suffer from vision problems.

For a variety of reasons, however, there will always be

some eye surgeons who routinely speak out against any pro-posed space-age advances in ophthalmic surgery. The ra-tionale behind these negative reactions varies widely and may often have nothing at all to do with the actual tools or tech-niques involved. Some ophthalmologists who do not possess the manual dexterity or the technical expertise that is necessary to utilize these new procedures, for example, may view the new technology and the dynamic younger surgeons who utilize it as a threat. Others, voicing a sincere but perhaps overly cautious opinion, may oppose what they view as the premature intro-duction of potentially dangerous techniques that they feel have not been studied fully.

This problem of opposition, however, should not be over-stated. At present, only the new techniques for refractive surgery are even somewhat in dispute; the modern high-tech methods of cataract extraction, as well as the various types of laser sur-gery used to treat other eye disorders, have all been generally accepted by the overall ophthalmic community.

Nonetheless, new ideas—especially those that are radi-cally different from current procedures—have a way of provok-ing controversy among physicians. The value of these develop-ments will be debated; some injuries and failures may initially occur. But ultimately, only those procedures that prove truly safe and effective will be offered to the general public.

It is therefore vitally important that we as eye-care patients remain as alert as possible to the development of new instru-ments and procedures. Once all of the proper studies on these experiments are completed and positive evaluations are re-ported, the public has the ability to loudly demand the best and most up-to-date treatment available. This is the only way to ensure that the concept of future vision will flourish.

AN EXCITING FUTURE LIES AHEAD

As we can learn by studying just a few of the experiments that are now being evaluated, an exciting future for the field of ophthalmology is very close at hand. We can see the amazing advances that have come about rapidly during the last few decades, and we can see the incredible developments that continue to occur almost every day. By looking at both the past and the present, we can almost envision what path eye surgery will take during the next few decades, even if the exact route remains somewhat of a mystery until we actually find ourselves there.

Thanks to recent developments in the field of high technology and the willingness of most eye surgeons to accept them, the prospects that are presented by today's ophthalmology are as exciting as any in medicine. But when we consider the almost unbelievable rate of scientific advancement that continues to take place right now, we can make only one sure prediction about the future of this medical specialty: Tomorrow's ophthalmology promises to be even better.

Think of that pre–World War II eye surgeon's journey into the 1980s, and then consider what a present-day ophthalmologist might learn from his colleagues in the future. While the exact specifications may be impossible to imagine, it is easy to see how we as patients will certainly continue to benefit.

10

Is Eye Surgery The Answer? How to Decide: Twelve Case Histories of Typical Eye Disorders

---

Thanks in part to its continuing introduction of new space-age tools and techniques, today's ophthalmology has created the tremendous surge in public optimism that now is associated with modern eye care. Not too many years ago, most of those who experienced a variety of common vision ailments knew that they would have to spend the rest of their lives with impaired eyesight. Now, many who suffer from these very same problems simply assume—often accurately—that some type of treatment already is available to correct them.

While it is true that certain eye problems still defy modern science, this growing public confidence definitely is well founded. In the last decade alone, a continuing series of ophthalmic innovations has turned our opinions on eye care upside down. We have learned that many "untreatable" vision disorders now can be cured through safe and simple operations. We have discovered that many "permanent" vision imperfections now can be corrected through painless and effective techniques. And, most importantly, we have determined that high technology now can allow us to retain a clear and accurate sense of vision for a lifetime.

One problem, however, is that today's ophthalmology has spawned a variety of technical terms and phrases that admittedly invite confusion. Devices like the cryolathe, YAG laser, potential acuity meter, intraocular lens implant, pachymeter, and diamond knife mean little to the uninformed. Procedures like phacoemulsification, iridotomy, keratomileusis, and trabeculoplasty offer little to the unaware. Those of us who are not ophthalmologists never should expect to understand them all, but by reading this book and then asking the right questions we still can benefit tremendously from the advances that these terms and phrases represent.

PUTTING KNOWLEDGE TO USE

Once we understand these tools and techniques, most of us then want to know how to put this knowledge to use. How can we decide when this new ophthalmic technology should be employed to correct our impaired eyesight? How can we judge which of the new techniques will be best to improve our failing vision? And how can we tell if eye surgery is right for our particular problem?

The ultimate answer, of course, can only come from a trained ophthalmologist. We may think we know what is causing our vision problem and we may be familiar with some of the modern techniques now being used to treat it. But we may not always be correct. It therefore is the ultimate responsibility of our eye physician—following a complete examination with the most accurate and up-to-date diagnostic tools available—to evaluate our problem and suggest the best conceivable solution.

It still is important, however, for the eye-care patient himself to know as much as possible about vision disorders and their modern treatments. Despite the existence of today's high-tech ophthalmic tools, no physician can diagnose a vision ailment properly unless the patient can outline all of the symptoms and problems that it has caused.

It is no longer a secret that most of the eye ailments discussed in this book offer clear and obvious symptoms that can be easily detected by any careful patient well *before* the problem leads to serious complications. The key to this early discovery is a very simple process, and one that we might call self-awareness.

Sometimes, however, self-awareness is mistakenly seen as self-diagnosis. Such untrained evaluation has never been encouraged by members of the medical profession, who reason that it can often prove more harmful than helpful. Many physicians claim that self-diagnosis can cause a patient to forego a regular medical checkup because his personal examination has not uncovered any problem worth pursuing. Or, they say, it may spark a needless fear of some sight- or even life-threatening illness that in reality does not even exist.

Granted, an absolute reliance on one's own untrained personal assessment of ambiguous signs or physical symptoms could cause a false sense of medical security. Just as seriously, it could lead to the use of dangerously ill-conceived folk treatments and potentially harmful home remedies. However, no responsible advocate of medical self-awareness would ever suggest that a patient rely totally upon his own self-evaluation. Rather, he will recommend this as merely one more tool in the important struggle for early detection and prompt treatment that is necessary to stop the spread of certain potential health problems.

A thorough knowledge of these disorders and treatments, then, can help the patient find an ophthalmologist who will understand his problem and recommend a solution that is safe, modern, and effective. Any patient who feels that his physician has unreasonably disagreed with his own assessment of the problem, or who believes that his physician irrationally has rejected a high-tech treatment for it, should seek a second opinion immediately.

Once again, though, the central question remains: How does a patient know when space-age eye surgery is the right solution for his own vision problem? Although no one really can answer this question without an accompanying eye exam, many of the most common eyesight disorders do offer a number of typical symptoms and preliminary characteristics that can give the observant patient an important first clue. When these clues are evaluated properly, they then can help to indicate whether today's high-tech surgical techniques might be utilized successfully to solve the patient's vision problem.

Listed below are a dozen sample scenarios that describe many of these common symptoms and characteristics often associated with the various eye disorders that are discussed in this book. They are followed by a simple explanation of the possible cause of these symptoms, as well as a notation if modern eye-surgical procedures might be useful in correcting the problem. Hopefully, these composite cases will be helpful to patients who are trying to decide if eye surgery will solve their own vision ailments.

Patient #1: Frank

Problem: Over the last several months, sixty-one-year-old Frank's vision has deteriorated gradually but steadily. Lately, he always thinks his glasses are dirty. He cannot see very well on bright days, and objects that he knows should be colorful instead look washed out or almost yellow.

Explanation: Symptoms such as these strongly indicate that Frank may be suffering from a cataract. He is in the proper age group, and a major clue is his gradual but steady onset of symptoms. Frank's "dirty glasses," trouble with bright light, and washed-out vision are all classic eyesight problems that often stem from the existence of a cataract. If an examination by an ophthalmologist confirms this diagnosis, a simple outpatient extraction, concluding with the implantation of an intraocular lens (IOL), will usually restore the patient's visual acuity to its previous high levels.

Patient #2: Ann

Problem: Ever since she was a little girl, Ann has been far-sighted. But now, at age twenty-seven, eyeglasses no longer seem to be capable of correcting her vision to acceptable levels. She tried wearing contact lenses once, but she just was never comfortable with them. (Her pair still is sitting in the medicine cabinet.) Ann wants to see the world as well as her friends do, and she is seeking a new alternative.

Explanation: While in the past all farsighted individuals such as Ann were resigned to wearing either eyeglasses or contact lenses, hyperopic keratomeleusis or HKM can now provide many of them with a third option. Under this safe and simple procedure, which is performed on an outpatient basis, the eye surgeon actually reshapes his patient's cornea so that it will be able to compensate for its natural inability to bend incoming light rays properly. If a thorough eye examination confirms Ann's self-diagnosis, it may be possible for a surgical correction to replace her old eyeglasses.

Patient #3: Richard

Problem: Richard, at age forty-six, had always considered himself to be a very lucky man as far as his eyesight was concerned—up to this stage in his life, he had never suffered from any vision problems at all. Lately, though, he has been noticing the gradual appearance of colored haloes around bright lights. He also believes that his side or peripheral vision is not as wide-ranging as it was in the past. Other than these two minor inconveniences, however, his eyesight seems to be as good as ever.

Explanation: Although it is impossible to tell for sure without a complete eye examination, Richard may be suffering from chronic open-angle glaucoma. The several related diseases that are generally known as glaucoma will strike about two percent of all people over age forty, and in its most common form—the one that Richard may have—it develops so gradually that it does not offer its victims many obvious symptoms. The two subtle vision problems that Richard has experienced, however, sometimes accompany the disease. If an eye examination indicates that Richard is indeed suffering from glaucoma, medication and a quick and painless laser treatment may prove to be the best way to reduce the chances of him losing his visual skills.

Patient #4: Carol

Problem: Carol, age sixty-three, has suffered from diabetes for almost twenty years. Although she has never experienced any major problems with her eyesight, lately it seems to her as if something is going on in her right eye. There has been some minor pain, and when she examines that eye in the mirror it just does not look right to her.

Explanation: Since Carol has been diabetic for nearly two decades, she most likely had been informed long ago of the need for regular eye examinations. Diabetics, especially those who have suffered from the disease for a number of years, are prone to diabetic retinopathy, which generally involves a breakdown in the structure, chemistry, or circulation of the eye's retina. While retinopathy can lead to blindness if not properly treated, eye surgeons today can utilize safe and efficient laser therapy to destroy the abnormal blood vessels that this disease tends to create.

Patient #5: Jim

Problem: Twenty-nine-year-old Jim is extremely near-sighted, so much so that he needs to wear his eyeglasses in the morning just to find his toothbrush. He has been bothered about the way his glasses affect his appearance ever since he was a youngster, but his vision is so poor that it has thus far proven impossible to fit him with acceptable contact lenses. Jim's lack of self-confidence keeps him from dating very often, and he spends most of his evenings alone in his apartment with his television or a book.

Explanation: Jim's painful lack of self-esteem may be related directly to his vision problems and the heavy glasses that are needed to correct it. If this is the case, he may be a good candidate for an outpatient surgical procedure called myopic keratomeleusis or MKM. This new and successful technique—in which an eye surgeon first removes a part of his patient's cornea and then reshapes it to correct his problem—may be Jim's best bet to continue life without the thick eyeglasses that seem to have caused him so much anguish. An ophthalmologist who is experienced in this technically demanding procedure should examine Jim further to determine whether MKM is a feasible means of correcting his vision impairment.

Patient #6: Rose

Problem: Something very strange has happened to the vision of fifty-nine-year-old Rose. At least as far as reading and knitting is concerned, her eyesight appears to be better than at any time in the past thirty years. The main problem with this improvement seems to be Rose's inability to get hold of a pair of eyeglasses that work—everytime she gets new ones, they have already become outdated for her ever-changing prescription.

Explanation: As suprising as it may sound, Rose's symptoms may indicate the presence of a cataract. As this common disorder gradually develops, the natural crystalline lens that is found in all eyes sometimes will change in a manner that actually seems to leave the patient more and more nearsighted. Since this change is continuous, the patient's prescriptions for eyeglasses will also become ineffective rather quickly. Although on the surface Rose's changes may sound beneficial, they most certainly are not if they are caused by a cataract. Vision loss will occur along with the apparent improvement, and a surgical cataract extraction is the only way that it can be reversed.

Patient #7: Norman

Problem: While he was watching TV in his den one night, fifty-three-year-old Norman suddenly saw what he thought was a flash of light in the lower portion of his left eye. A few minutes later, he saw it again. For the rest of the evening Norman tried to catch the light flash, but it never seemed to occur when he was paying attention. As soon as his mind moved on to other things, however, the flash of light reappeared.

Explanation: Norman's light flashes—and associated "floaters"—are one of the classic symptoms of a retinal tear. This potentially serious problem is most common among those between the ages of fifty and sixty and can lead to retinal detachment and eventual blindness. A detachment occurs when the eye's retina pulls away from its adjoining layer, and it may result from a blow to the eye, some other type of disease, or simply as a natural consequence of the aging process. Left untreated, a retinal detachment can lead to blindness, but symptoms such as Norman's are a good indication that it is time for the patient to seek medical care. Modern laser therapy, performed on an outpatient basis, often can repair the holes and tears that will lead to such a detachment even before it occurs.

Patient #8: Deborah

Problem: When forty-nine-year-old Deborah received a telephone call informing her that her best friend from childhood had been killed in a car crash, she went into a deep and immediate emotional depression. A few moments later she developed the most severe headache that she had ever experienced, as well as a violent case of nausea that was accompanied by constant vomiting. At first Deborah thought the symptoms were related entirely to her grief, but when she noticed that her vision was becoming blurred and the lights in her bedroom seemed to be surrounded by colored haloes, she suspected that something else might be wrong.

Explanation: While the headache and nausea alone might stem solely from Deborah's intense grief, the vision problems that accompanied them are a strong indication that something else had indeed gone wrong. From her description, it sounds as if Deborah may be suffering from acute angle-closure glaucoma, which is an extremely serious but relatively uncommon form of this eye disease. Unlike other variations of glaucoma, this form can develop quickly and unexpectedly among certain patients whose pupils suddenly dilate very widely as a result of emotional stress, severe pain, certain drugs, or other causes. Unless this condition is relieved promptly by surgical means, blindness can occur in only a day or two.

Patient #9: Sam

Problem: At the age of eighty-four, Sam's greatest pleasure in life is his daily habit of reading the morning newspaper while seated on a wooden bench in the park near his home. In recent weeks, however, he has had more and more trouble reading the paper. At first he suspected that the newspaper's publishers had altered the size or the style of their typeface, but when he called them about it they denied any change. He then began to wonder if, after all these years, his prescription had worsened and he would need new eyeglasses.

Explanation: Sam's problem may have its cause in his eyeglass prescription, but it also may be due to an eye disorder called macular degeneration. In its most common form, macular degeneration is found most often among the elderly, and while it rarely leads to blindness the disease can severely affect the patient's central or reading vision. This disorder stems from changes that occur in the center of the eye's retina, beginning with small hemorrhages and continuing with the development of abnormal blood vessels. In certain cases, macular degeneration can be treated successfully by means of outpatient laser therapy. But only a complete eye examination by a qualified physician can determine whether this treatment will be successful.

Patient #10: Audrey

Problem: Audrey, thirty-seven years old, suffers from a relatively moderate case of nearsightedness that requires her to wear her prescription lenses in order to drive, read, and work. Since she secured a new job at the local coal mine, however, she has found her existing lenses now pose a number of troublesome problems. Audrey's trusty eyeglasses constantly get scratched from flying debris or they slip out of place from the sweat on her nose. If she tries to wear her contact lenses in the mine's dust-filled environment, they constantly irritate her eyes.

Explanation: Audrey sounds as if she may be a perfect candidate for radial keratotomy or RK, which can be used to surgically correct certain low levels of nearsightedness. Audrey seems to have all of the right reasons for considering this proven surgical alternative—a prescription and age that fall within required limits, and a justifiable inability to continue wearing her old eyeglasses or contact lenses. If an ophthalmologist's examination confirms her suitability for this technique, Audrey may be able to put her glasses and contacts away forever.

Patient #11: Albert

Problem: Seventy-year-old Albert knows he is suffering from a cataract, but he is not certain whether it is time to have it removed yet. He still can drive, but only if the sun is not too bright. He still can read, but only if he squeezes his bad eye tightly shut. And since Albert is retired, the only other inconvenience that he experiences is the blurry haze that envelops objects that are about thirty feet or so away from him.

Explanation: Albert is correct—he does have a cataract—and it *is* hard to know for sure whether now is the time to have it removed. The most difficult decision that anyone suffering from cataracts must make is when an extraction should be scheduled, and despite all of today's diagnostic tools, this decision only can be made by the patient himself. There are some common guidelines that often are used to help make this decision, however, and the most important of all concerns the cataract's impact on the patient's lifestyle. Albert is having some trouble driving, reading, and even seeing across the street. It therefore is probably a good time for his cataract to be removed.

Patient #12: Sophia

Problem: Sophia, age sixty-six, was telling her brother about a number of "minor" eye problems that she had been experiencing. She told him that her vision seemed distorted, that there was some pain in her eyes, and that her eyelids sometimes looked as if they were swollen. She also told him that she could not remember the last time she had visited an ophthalmologist.

Explanation: While Sophia's symptoms could point to the existence of several serious eye disorders, nothing definite can be determined without a thorough—and apparently long-overdue—eye exam. Periodic examinations by a qualified eye physician are an important part of maintaining good health as we grow older. Early detection of the various visual problems that are associated with aging often is the only sure way to prevent permanent eyesight loss. Most ophthalmologists recommend that those aged forty and older undergo a complete eye exam every two to five years. High-risk individuals—those with diabetes or a family history of such problems as glaucoma, cataracts, or retinal detachment—should seek more frequent care. And anyone who experiences any of the symptoms like those described in this chapter should schedule an immediate visit with their ophthalmologist.

11

Paying For Eye Care

As the twentieth century draws to a close, there can be no denying that health care has become very expensive, and it is getting more so all the time. Some say the general inflationary trend of our economy is a chief reason for this state of affairs. Others insist that it stems primarily from the necessary but costly experimentation that results in dramatic new medical advances. A third group places the blame squarely upon those fully insured patients who seek medical care with no regard to cost. And still another group attributes the problem completely to all health-care providers who do not wish to offer 1980 services at 1950 prices.

While it is difficult to pinpoint the exact source of the problem, most observers agree that it more than likely comes from a complicated combination of each one of these causes. And, if that is the case, all of them must be examined as a part of the solution.

A REAL CRISIS EXISTS

The very idea that a serious health-care crisis does exist in this country is no longer open to debate. Health care has become the third largest industry in the United States, with today's total annual medical tab of several hundred billion dollars expected to top the one trillion mark by 1990. Even by the mid-1980s, however, health-care expenditures already were rising twice as fast as the Consumer Price Index and had amounted to more than 12 percent of the nation's Gross National Product.

Unfortunately, the nation's continually rising medical bills arrived at a time when a number of its citizens were increasingly unable to pay. While the country's elderly population—those who experience the vast majority of costly, chronic illnesses—grows considerably larger each year, their incomes and expenses move farther apart. Elderly Americans, for example, now often find that their health-care bills represent a painfully large portion of their entire annual income.

None of this, of course, should be allowed to have any bearing on the eventual delivery of health-care services to the people who most need them. We are at a point in our history when continuing medical developments offer new hope to many patients who might previously have had none. It therefore is ironic—and totally unfair—when many of these advances are not utilized only because a patient feels that he cannot afford the resulting bills. Avoidable blindness that results solely from a patient's lack of financial resources is a disease of society that is far worse than the actual vision impairment that caused it.

While nearly everyone would agree that this situation should not be permitted, it is already too much of a reality. We all have heard the joke about the hospital admittance clerk who requires a pregnant woman to completely fill out her insurance forms, even as she is going into obvious labor. While this story may exaggerate the truth to some extent, the problem that it represents most certainly is real. As the health-care industry continually shifts from an ignore-the-cost attitude to a reduce-the-cost imperative, it moves ever closer to the possibility that only those patients who can afford medical care will be able to obtain it.

Thankfully, that day has not yet arrived. Most Americans are covered by some type of medical insurance, either government or private, and they still can rely on these programs to pay at least a portion of their health-care bills. But even many of those who lack adequate insurance coverage still can obtain necessary treatment through a substantial number of charitable medical practitioners and subsidized public hospitals.

THE GOVERNMENT FOOTS THE BILL

The overwhelming majority of America's health-care bills, in fact, are paid by government funds. This hardly is surprising when one considers that most of the nation's elderly and many of its disabled are eligible for the federal Medicare program, while millions more are eligible for the indigent care that is provided by the combination federal-state program known as Medicaid. The billing for these two government efforts alone accounts for nearly half of every health-care dollar that is spent today.

As both health-care costs and the government's contribution to them continued their meteoric rise during the early 1980s, however, the potential for economic disaster loomed large and a movement toward reform was begun. Because public officials are under constant pressure to trim costs, many looked toward the growing expenses that were related to the government's medical programs. While it was generally agreed that these programs were necessary to the nation's well-being, it also was argued that immediate action must be initiated. Some considered limiting federal contributions; others pondered cutting the programs out entirely.

Horrified by the thought of trimming or eliminating such critical programs with proven worth, saner heads responded with a compromise proposal. Under it, the government actually would use Medicare, the nation's single largest provider of health-care coverage, in an attempt to stem the cost-increase tide. The resulting 1983 DRG program (for *diagnosis-related group*) required the government to first determine how much a number of common medical services should cost, and then to reimburse health care providers only that amount for performing these procedures. Many private insurance companies soon followed Medicare's lead, and DRG quickly became the medical buzzword of the decade.

PRIVATE PROVIDERS FOLLOWED SUIT

The next move came from health-care providers themselves. Prodded by simple economics, a number of these providers—just as Medicare officials had predicted—then cut the fees that they charged for certain services to the amount that insurance companies would cover. While the jury still is out on the ultimate effect of this program, it has been subject thus far to criticism as well as commendation. Some attribute the effort to slowing the increase in medical costs, for example, while others claim it only is responsible for premature hospital releases and cutbacks in needed care.

Whatever the final verdict, the impact of DRGs has already been significant. One initial result was the widespread movement toward outpatient surgery. Another was the controversial establishment of *peer-review organizations* (PROs), which are designed to review the necessity, quality, and cost of Medicare services before they are administered. Like the DRGs themselves, these two efforts have gathered both critics and supporters.

Additional responses to the cost-cutting frenzy that is now prevalent in health care have centered on the establishment and growth of so-called *alternative delivery systems.* These new efforts, which attempt to provide an option to traditional fee-for-service private physicians, include such alphabet soup—nicknamed programs as the health maintenance organization (HMO), preferred provider organization (PPO), and individual practice association (IPA). While some of these programs have been in existence for a decade or more, they were so small until the advent of DRGs that their effectiveness, too, cannot yet be assessed adequately.

While it is still too early to tell whether any of these alternatives will have a beneficial long-term effect on health-care costs, they certainly have offered the patient a variety of new options. Today's health-care programs allow the patient to pick and choose from among a variety of diverse coverage plans, which enables him to select a program that best fits his medical needs and personal lifestyle. Unfortunately, many of these new plans continue to look at basic medical coverage in the same tired old way as their predecessors, and so their options may not provide such an alternative after all.

COVERAGE GAPS STILL EXIST

Most insurance programs, old and new, will fund the treatment of a diagnosed illness, for example, but they will not pay for regular medical checkups or so-called preventive care. Since it is recognized widely today that early diagnosis is often the only way to prevent certain problems, including a number of common vision disorders, it certainly seems counterproductive to discourage patients from checkups by refusing to pay for them unless a disease is uncovered. Perhaps that, too, will change.

For the present, however, eye care is funded by public and private insurance companies in much the same manner as treatment in other medical specialties is covered. Unless it is expressly provided by a particular policy, for example, regular checkups are paid for only if some type of disease is found. After the diagnosis of an illness, however, all prescribed treatment generally is covered to some extent (anywhere from 80 to 100 percent of the total cost).

While private insurance usually is more comprehensive than Medicare, there often are important gaps in both coverage plans that should be recognized by the patient. Medicare, for example, will not cover routine office visits or any auxiliary items such as eyeglasses or prescription drugs. Most private insurance plans also will not cover these items, although some of the better programs now are beginning to offer far more extensive funding practices in an effort to remain competitive. Those who are unfamiliar with their policies should check them as thoroughly as possible beforehand, so there will be no surprises when a bill is submitted for payment.

QUESTIONS ABOUT COVERAGE

Patients who still do not understand their coverage should ask questions before any treatment is undertaken. For those with private insurance, the first place to turn usually is the policy administrator. For those with government insurance and those with remaining concerns, the best source of information will be the billing personnel in your ophthalmologist's office. These knowledgable people are accustomed to dealing with Medicare and a variety of private programs, and they almost always can answer your questions about what is covered and what is not.

If a patient requires treatment and has inadequate insurance—or even no insurance at all—the ophthalmologist's billing office still is a good place to go and ask for help. Often, personnel in these offices will be more than willing to arrange some type of acceptable payment plan so that nobody will be forced to forego needed treatment solely for financial reasons. It is critical, however, that such alternative payment plans always be arranged *in advance of all medical care* and not after those services are rendered. Most physicians are willing to work with their patients on payment options, but only if the matter is discussed prior to treatment.

Although in today's constantly changing environment it is not feasible to provide a comprehensive, up-to-date outline of the ophthalmic coverage that is offered by Medicare and all of the nation's private insurance companies, it is possible to discuss the manner in which the space-age techniques that are described in this book typically are funded. Since the amount of payment and the manner in which it is obtained can vary significantly from state to state and from procedure to procedure, however, it is important for the patient to obtain precise information on his policy if any questions remain.

SOME GENERAL RULES APPLY

A few general funding rules apply to all of the various ophthalmic procedures discussed in this book. First, as was indicated earlier, only a few private insurance plans will cover routine eye examinations—unless an illness is detected, in which case the exam and all subsequent treatment is usually covered. Second, since outpatient surgery is encouraged these days by nearly all insurance programs, some may offer increased payment when this option is utilized in a state-licensed or Medicare-approved facility.

Next, most private insurance companies will offer larger payments than Medicare after their specified deductibles are met, although an adequately insured patient rarely will be responsible for more than 20 percent of his entire bill. And finally, the Medicare patient who also can afford to carry some type of supplemental private insurance almost always can expect to receive the fullest and most complete coverage.

As perhaps the most common and successful of all high-tech ophthalmic procedures, cataract surgery is covered at least partially by practically every insurance program that is available today. Because most programs now set an *allowable* or *approved* rate for cataract removal, these plans do not differentiate between intracapsular extraction, extracapsular extraction, and phacoemulsification; they simply offer a set payment for the procedure no matter how it is performed. The implantation of an intraocular lens immediately following cataract surgery or at any time thereafter also is at least partially covered by most programs.

Since it also has evolved into a proven and commonplace technique, most insurance companies now offer excellent coverage for nearly all types of laser surgery when it has been prescribed for a vision disorder. This includes argon and neodymium-YAG laser therapy for glaucoma or various retinal problems, as well as the laser treatment often employed for the aftereffects of some cataract extractions. When the procedure is medically necessary and performed in an outpatient setting, in fact, many insurance programs will now pay the entire approved amount.

Since refractive surgery to correct nearsightedness, farsightedness, and astigmatism almost never is performed on Medicare patients (because it is most beneficial to a much younger age group), these procedures generally are paid for only by certain private insurance companies which specify such coverage in their policies. If there is a legitimate reason for undergoing refractive surgery—such as an inability to wear eyeglasses or contact lenses due to physical, emotional, or occupational factors—the chance for receiving full or partial payment is greatly enhanced. When appropriate, ophthalmologists will submit written verification to the insurance carrier noting that such surgery is not being performed for cosmetic purposes.

Claim Submittal is Easy

The actual submission of surgery claims to government and private insurance carriers may be the easiest part of the entire process. At the time such surgery is initially scheduled, most patients will be asked to meet with the ophthalmologist's billing personnel. These professionals then will take down the patient's insurance information and immediately inform him how much of the procedure's cost will be covered. If the patient is confused or dissatisfied with his coverage, he still has time to check into the matter further before surgery day.

Unless there is a dispute, from that point on the surgical patient usually will have nothing else to do with the insurance process. The billing office generally will handle all of the remaining paperwork, including the actual filing of the claim. However, patients with some types of private insurance may need to bring in their own claim forms in order to insure their total coverage. (Although a generic *universal claim form* can be filed, certain insurance companies require that their clients initiate all claims on company forms; these, too, can be filled out and submitted by the billing office personnel.)

Following surgery, the ophthalmologist will receive payment directly from the insurance company, with the exact amount determined by the patient's specific coverage. If only partial payment was provided, most patients then will receive a bill for the difference. However, federal law specifies that all Medicare patients who are able to demonstrate financial hardship must have their cases reviewed individually by the ophthalmologist involved. After such a review, the eye surgeon may choose not to require that his patient pay anything additional.

FUNDING SHOULD NOT AFFECT CARE

Like all forms of health care today, there is no doubt that proper eye care can prove to be very expensive. But the alternative—impaired vision or even total blindness—certainly is a much more painful option. And in this day and age, when the new space-age ophthalmic tools and techniques that now are available have been developed to a level never before thought possible, it would be particularly sad to allow funding worries to get in the way of necessary treatment.

This does not *have* to happen, and it should not be allowed to occur. Insurance coverage, for the most part, has responded to the changes in medicine and most of today's high-tech surgical procedures now are at least partially funded by the majority of reputable companies. And many private physicians and health-care institutions will work along with their needy, underinsured patients in order to provide them with the medical care that they require.

If a vision problem does occur, there is no longer any excuse for not investigating what today's ophthalmology can do to treat it. In many cases, the advances in ophthalmic tools and techniques that have appeared during the last decade now mean that blindness often can be prevented, but only when the patient takes the initiative to do so.

12

How to Choose an Eye Surgeon

Without question, our basic concept of eye care today is dramatically different than it was even a decade ago. Because of new high-tech procedures employed by a growing number of ophthalmic surgeons, many eye diseases and vision disorders that once were considered untreatable now can be safely and effectively corrected in an outpatient facility. These advances have improved the treatment for so many common eye ailments, in fact, that for the first time in history most of us legitimately can expect to spend our entire lifetimes with clear and unimpaired eyesight.

Despite the mind-boggling advances that have been made in the field of ophthalmology, however, it still is the patient who holds the greatest responsibility for his own vision health. He must, for example, schedule regular eye examinations, which often are the only way to catch a potentially sight-threatening disease such as glaucoma before extensive and irreversible damage has been done. And he must constantly be alert for any signs or symptoms of trouble, which can help an ophthalmologist to correctly and timely diagnose his disorder.

But the patient also has another vitally important responsibility once it has been determined that a vision problem actually exists. If the ailment is one of the many that can be corrected by using today's modern surgical techniques, he must select an eye surgeon who is adequately trained and experienced in these space-age procedures. Unless the precision tools and demanding techniques of the new ophthalmology are in the proper hands, they will not do anyone any good.

PROPER SELECTION IS CRITICAL

The choice of a qualified eye surgeon can offer a variety of challenges—particularly to those who do not already have a regular ophthalmologist of their own—but the proper selection is critical to any operation's eventual success as well as the patient's peace of mind. By following a few simple preliminary investigatory steps and by carefully and deliberately questioning the prospective surgeon, however, anyone can select a trustworthy ophthalmologist who is trained and experienced in these modern procedures.

The first step for any patient who has been informed of a need for eye surgery is to gather as much information as possible about his particular vision problem. Next, he should learn as much as he can about the expertise that the diagnosing physician has amassed in this area. Finally, he should find out whether his ophthalmologist is experienced in the field's new high-tech procedures. Only after all of these issues have been resolved will the patient feel entirely confident about the operation that he is about to face.

As the search for an eye surgeon begins, it is important for the patient to initially recognize the different types of vision specialists that are available today and to fully understand the services that each can provide. *Ophthalmologist* is often used interchangeably with *eye surgeon,* and that is because this medical doctor is the only type of eye specialist qualified to both diagnose and treat diseases and defects of the eye. Ophthalmologists are trained to perform eye surgery, measure changes of vision, determine whether one is nearsighted or farsighted, and prescribe corrective lenses. Therefore, only an ophthalmologist can perform the sight-saving procedures that are described in this book.

Some ophthalmologists also concentrate on a subspecialty, and by focusing on a particular area they often will be the most qualified to treat that type of vision disorder. A specialist such as a corneal surgeon, retinal surgeon, or cataract surgeon usually has received one or two years of additional training in the treatment of that specific disease or component of the eye, and he probably spends a major portion of his operating time on patients with that ailment. Nonetheless, a subspeciality alone does not guarantee any expertise in today's high-tech procedures.

Before a patient can decide whether or not to choose a specialist, he must first fully examine that physician's practice. For example, there are cataract surgeons who acquired their specialty credentials many years ago but now perform only a few such operations annually. And there also are cataract surgeons who use the latest space-age extraction techniques but still do not inspire much confidence among their patients. If one or both of these situations is encountered, the careful patient will be wise to continue his physician search.

The central issues, obviously, are trust and expertise. Most patients want an eye surgeon with whom they can feel comfortable, as well as one who knows about the latest treatments that can be used for their particular vision disorder. If the patient hopes to have his ailment corrected safely and effectively, therefore, he must locate an ophthalmologist who has both the training and the experience necessary to use today's high-tech tools and techniques in a humane and compassionate manner.

Locating a Surgeon

There are a number of ways for a patient to locate such a specially trained ophthalmologist, even within an unfamiliar geographic area. If an eye surgeon is the one who first diagnosed the problem that is in need of attention and the patient determines after investigation that this physician has the expertise to perform the procedure, he may be the best option of all. This physician already is familiar with the patient and his disorder, and if the patient feels comfortable with him, there is little reason to look elsewhere.

If the diagnosing ophthalmologist says he is not qualified to perform the needed surgery or the patient is not confident in his surgical abilities, however, it will be necessary to select another surgeon. This can be accomplished in a variety of ways, all of which involve questioning other physicians as well as patients with similar vision problems, and then talking to the prospective eye surgeon himself.

If the patient is in his home area, the first step can be to ask a trusted family doctor for a few recommendations. Since vision problems are fairly common, especially those discussed in this book, most family practitioners will have encountered them before and therefore should be able to suggest a good operating ophthalmologist. But even a top-notch family doctor may not be aware of all the eye surgeons in his community, and he may not be familiar with the ones who can perform today's high-tech procedures. So while this step may provide some good initial possibilities, the patient also should seek out other candidates before the search is concluded.

Two ways that this can be done, even in a strange town, are by checking with the local medical society or the head ophthalmologist at the local hospital. Each of these options, however, has drawbacks as well as advantages. Medical societies, for example, usually will recommend only those physicians who have paid dues to join their group. And head ophthalmologists usually are very busy and hard to reach. Nonetheless, either of these options may provide the patient with a list of excellent surgeons who are experienced in treating their specific problem.

The government, too, often can prove helpful to the patient who is attempting to locate an eye surgeon. Federal officials operate a toll-free Second Opinion Hotline (1-800-638-

6833; or in Maryland, 1-800-492-6603) that offers information that may prove helpful to those seeking a specialist in any geographical area. Patients covered by Medicare can contact their local Social Security office (which will be listed in the telephone directory under "U.S. Government, Department of Health, Education, and Welfare"). Medicaid patients can contact their local welfare office.

If the patient is in or near his hometown, the search can be simplified greatly by asking for suggestions from friends, relatives, or neighbors who previously have undergone the same operation. The patient, however, always should consider the qualifications of the person who is offering the recommendation. Are they reliable? Have their past recommendations usually proven acceptable? Is the physician that they are suggesting fully trained and experienced in the right area? If the answer to these questions is "yes," this type of recommendation almost always can prove to be best.

A final way to obtain an eye surgeon, particularly in a town where none of the above methods can be employed, is through the many advertisements that now appear on television or in local newspapers and telephone directories. Since these ads usually are produced by the physician or an agency that he has hired, they may provide an excellent starting point but the patient should never rely on them alone. Just as he should do with verbal recommendations, the patient should question these advertising ophthalmologists in person and perhaps ask to speak with a few former patients who have undergone treatment for the same disorder.

The Patient Must Be Comfortable

Asking questions is, in fact, an excellent idea even for those patients who are familiar with their ophthalmologist. Before agreeing to any elective eye surgery—or any type of nonemergency surgery, for that matter—the patient should be certain that the recommended procedure really is necessary at that time. The patient should understand what is wrong with him, what type of surgery has been suggested, what the benefits and risks of this operation will be, how long recovery will take, how much the procedure costs and whether it is covered by insurance, and what will happen if the patient does not schedule surgery.

If the patient is uncomfortable with the answers to any of these questions, it is a good idea for him to seek a second opinion from another qualified doctor. Most eye surgeries are elective, nonemergency procedures that usually are scheduled far in advance, so there generally is plenty of time to obtain this additional advice. A second opinion is standard medical procedure, often covered by private and government insurance policies, and should not be considered an outright rejection of the first physician's diagnosis. Together with that initial recommendation, however, it may help to convince the skeptical patient whether surgery is absolutely necessary or can be postponed.

Finding a surgeon for a second opinion can be accomplished in the same manner as finding a primary ophthalmologist. When this second opinion finally is obtained, the patient should tell the physician about any diagnostic tests that already were performed as well as the type of surgery that was recommended. If this doctor agrees that the surgery is necessary, it generally is best for the patient to go back to the first ophthalmologist, who already is familiar with his problem and his eyes, for treatment.

If the second doctor disagrees, however, the patient is faced with a difficult dilemma. He may go back to the first physician to discuss his problem further, seek the opinion of a third ophthalmologist, or weigh the two conflicting opinions that he already has obtained and make up his own mind. It is important for the patient to remember that qualified physicians who examine the same eyes may still disagree on a course of treatment, and in many cases both may present valid arguments to prove their point. It therefore is critical that the patient himself be totally confident with the course of action that he eventually chooses.

Watch Out For Phonies

While it may seem obvious to stress that only an eye surgeon is able to treat the various vision disorders that are discussed in this book, today's society is plagued by phony cures that are offered by medical quacks who prey on those who most need health care. These dishonest promoters regularly make a number of outrageous claims through a variety of printed advertisements, and they are able to lure unsuspecting patients into spending a good deal of money for items that will eventually prove totally useless.

Everyone should resist the urge to purchase a mail-order "miracle product" that promises a "quick and painless cure" through the application of some "secret formula." If something sounds too good to be true, it usually is. Before sending any money for such an item, prospective purchasers first should check it out with a trusted physician, their local consumer-affairs office, or the Better Business Bureau. And they should keep in mind what has often been said in this book. When eye care is concerned, only an ophthalmologist is qualified to treat vision diseases and disorders.

Aided as they have been by the advances in tools and techniques that have appeared over the last decade or so, today's ophthalmologist is truly a high-tech scientist who is meeting the needs of our space-age society. Now, we not only are experiencing a longer lifetime than any generation before us, but thanks to a number of medical developments, we also are living these lives more completely than our forefathers. Modern eye surgeons have played a critical role in this development and they probably will play an even greater part as newer and better advances are introduced in the coming years.

AN ACTIVE ROLE IS VITAL

It still remains vitally important that we all continue to take an active role in our overall health, however, which means that we must become knowledgable and cautious consumers of all types of medical care. This includes eye care, of course, where we not only must be aware of early signs and symptoms that will help us to pinpoint a vision disorder before it becomes serious, but also in the way that we actually choose our vision-treatment specialist.

While most ophthalmologists are able to surgically treat glaucoma or successfully remove a cataract, for example, not everyone can perform these procedures with the most modern and up-to-date techniques that are available today. And while most of the older techniques certainly have proven themselves over time as safe and effective treatments for a given vision impairment, many of them simply are no match for the new developments which offer even safer and more effective alternatives.

In addition, there is one important area—refractive surgery—that is still relatively new. Some ophthalmologists have expressed concern that long-term consequences for these innovative techniques have not yet been fully investigated and they therefore advise their patients to avoid them. In reality, however, many hundreds of thousands of these operations already have been performed on satisfied patients throughout the world and a knowledgable health care consumer will be able to sort out the available evidence and make up his own mind as to the viability of these procedures.

Considering the great possibilities that lay before us—as well as the tremendous roadblocks that can conspire against us—it is critical that we as patients take an increasingly active role in our vision care. We may not be able to heal ourselves, but there is other action that we can take which will have just as big an impact. Primarily, this means the practice of preventive eye care and the careful selection of a vision specialist.

When an eye disease or vision disorder does strike, it is important that we select an eye surgeon who not only makes us feel comfortable, but who is also experienced in the most modern and effective treatment methods yet developed. Only then will we be assured of getting the best care available, and only then will the promises of future vision be fulfilled.

13

Rewards of Being a Space-Age Ophthalmologist

Few other fields of medicine have come to rely on space-age technology as completely as ophthalmology. A visit to an eye doctor's examining room today is like a trip into the future, and its benefits can be just as exciting for those who suffer from visual impairment as for those who attempt to cure them.

Early ophthalmologists were severely limited in their mission by the inherent difficulty of examining and repairing a spherical object that is less than an inch in diameter. Even as recently as the turn of the twentieth century, in fact, most ophthalmic instruments were so crude that eye surgeons literally could not always see what they were trying to do. The cause and development of cataracts, refractive errors, glaucoma, and retinal disorders has been somewhat understood for many decades, but tools and techniques of the past seriously limited the type of surgical procedures that could be used to rectify them.

This limitation is the reason why so many ailments now considered minor were often left uncorrected, and why others had to be treated with a variety of primitive techniques that proved only partially effective. It was not until recent technological advances permitted ophthalmologists to first see the eye better, and then to develop the type of miniaturized tools necessary to work within it, that eye surgery was able to leap beyond the constraints that had held it back for hundreds of years.

ADVANCES STEM FROM DEDICATION

Of course, none of these breakthroughs would have occurred without the dedication and perserverance of today's eye surgeons. Always seeking better avenues of treatment for common vision problems, ophthalmic researchers throughout the world have been responsible for the many new tools and techniques that can now be routinely used to save our sight. And while many of today's developments seem to depend entirely upon such space-age machines as the laser and cryolathe, none could be performed without the competent guidance of a trained ophthalmologist.

The eye surgeons who support and utilize this new technology far outnumber those who do not, and their ranks are growing larger all the time. Ophthalmologists in general now recognize that most of these space-age tools and techniques will provide them with the best way to help their patients, and the majority are therefore enthusiastic about employing them.

To a really good surgeon, top-notch medical care will always remain the highest priority. This is the reason why so many American doctors will voluntarily shut down their practices to temporarily head for places like the U.S.S.R., Mexico, and various Third World countries that desperately need humanitarian care and free medical support. And since they will only be in these nations for a few days at most, the physicians must work around the clock, with no financial compensation, to provide needed treatment to a populace literally starved for modern health care.

Despite today's popularly held public perception, most physicians have not entered the profession for the money that it can bring them. Most practice medicine because they have a deep concern for people.

UTILIZING MODERN TECHNIQUES

In order to most successfully help those who suffer from eye problems today, it is absolutely necessary that the tools and techniques introduced in recent years be utilized to their fullest. Modern ophthalmologists *must* be prepared to perform state-of-the-art cataract surgery with an intraocular lens implantation. They *must* be skilled in techniques of laser surgery. They *must* be aware of the various surgical alternatives to eyeglasses and contact lenses. And they *must* be willing to perform these high-tech procedures in an outpatient setting.

Those physicians who accept the possibilities and potentials of the new ophthalmology will certainly reap greater rewards and satisfactions than those who do not. Offering vision to a needlessly sightless patient will always be one of the truly great feelings that an eye surgeon can obtain; doing so by means of the safest, most painless method available intensifies these feelings.

Ophthalmologists who have entered the profession in recent decades have found themselves participating in a brave new world of eye surgery. They must possess a very high degree of manual dexterity as well as a desire to work with complicated high-tech machinery. They must be willing to accept the fact that today's state-of-the-art procedures can change completely overnight, as well as the fact that today's patients are generally more knowledgable about medical options and the treatments they are about to receive.

OPHTHALMOLOGY HAS ALWAYS BEEN AN APPEALING SPECIALTY

For a variety of reasons, ophthalmology has always proven to be an appealing field for aspiring doctors. First, it offers an exciting opportunity to pursue fine surgical skills. Second, it offers a rare opportunity to diagnose a problem and then surgically correct it. Third, it offers a rewarding opportunity to often spot certain serious ailments, such as hypertension and diabetes, before other types of physicians can find it and before any related damage has been done.

But finally—and perhaps more importantly—the vast majority of ophthalmic patients are actually quite healthy. Unlike some other medical specialties, the pain and suffering that stems from vision impairment or eye disease can often be completely alleviated in the operating room. The endless scenario of death and dying that physicians who are practicing in other branches of medicine must confront on a daily basis is nonexistent.

Nonetheless, ophthalmology remained a relatively uncrowded profession as recently as the late 1970s. Despite the advances that had occurred and were continuing to occur at that time, the field was still mostly mired in the Dark Ages.

Of course, there were some exceptions among both practicing ophthalmologists and those who were studying to join their ranks. Several fine programs—such as the ones at New York City's Manhattan Eye, Ear, and Throat Hospital, UCLA's Jules Stein Eye Institute, Philadelphia's Wills Eye Institute, Houston's Baylor University, the University of Iowa, and the University of Illinois—attracted flocks of future space-age ophthalmologists by providing their young surgical residents with an excellent exposure to the changing world of eye surgery.

However, a number of other programs did not focus on the new high-tech ophthalmic techniques at all, and many of these also assigned the bulk of their surgical cases to affiliated surgical fellows. This unfortunate practice offered eager residents little more than the opportunity to observe the performance of outdated surgical procedures, and it may therefore have ended up turning some excellent, but increasingly frustrated, young medical students away from the field of ophthalmology.

AN OPHTHALMOLOGICAL EDUCATION

The training of an ophthalmologist is a lengthy and difficult process that begins immediately after college when the prospective physician first attends four years of medical school and then completes his surgically oriented internship. This initial medical education is quite general in nature and is not tied to any particular medical specialty, however, so it is not until the three-year ophthalmic residency that follows that the detailed techniques and terminology of vision treatment will be taught.

Since the new resident has thus far received only minimal training in the workings of the eye, his first year begins with an introduction to its basics. While the ophthalmic resident is completing formal course work, he will also learn how to test a patient's vision and be introduced to the equipment that is necessary to perform such examinations. He will also observe eye surgery for perhaps the first time, and possibly assist the attending staff with certain procedures.

The majority of prospective physicians who have gotten this far in the medical-education process will eventually go on to become practicing ophthalmologists. Because of the extremely high motivation of most students who have reached this level, as well as the strict screening process that most ophthalmic programs are forced to employ—the number of applicants is much higher than the number of openings—the dropout rate is virtually zero from this point on.

During the second year, the resident will begin work in several new areas of ophthalmic microsurgery such as reconstructive plastic surgery around the eyes and eyelids, and eye muscle surgery. This middle segment of an ophthalmic resident's education contains a good deal more hands-on surgical training than did the previous year, and much of the work is actually performed on real patients. (Many medical schools offer free or low-cost care to those patients who are willing to be examined and treated by one of their residents.)

At this time, many of the second-year residents will additionally receive their first intensive introduction to the tools and techniques of space-age eye surgery by undergoing some initial specialty training in areas like the retina and the use of ophthalmic lasers. In top programs like those mentioned earlier, the young physician will also be offered the chance to actually use this knowledge in real surgical situations.

In the third and final year, a resident will be taught the basics of intraocular lens implantation technique and begin to operate on cataracts. He will also learn about other, less common surgical procedures, such as corneal transplants, that have not yet been discussed. At this time, the resident may also select an area of ophthalmology in which he wishes to specialize.

Following his three-year residency, the physician will graduate as an ophthalmologist. In order to become a specialist in certain areas such as the retina, the physician will need to pursue a fellowship and study further. Most others will attempt to obtain board certification within two years of completing their residency. (While recognized by the public as a minimum level of expertise required for ophthalmic surgeons, such certification is not required and some ophthalmologists elect not to obtain it.)

Even for those who formally begin their medical practice at this time, however, the educational process is not complete. In fact, it will never be totally complete for any top-level surgeon. Due primarily to today's rapid and consistent developments in all fields of medicine, in a given number of years even the most accomplished physician will find that his technical knowledge has become outdated. It is therefore critical that all physicians go on to secure so-called *continuing medical education* credits (CME) at various regularly scheduled seminars and training sessions. Ophthalmologists who specialize in space-age surgery often attend special sessions several times each year that are taught by the originators of these high-tech tools and procedures.

It is generally recognized that this intricate but informal "tutoring system," as well as its members' continuing quest for newer and better surgical technology and techniques, sets today's good eye surgeons apart from the great ones.

TODAY'S EYE-CARE REVOLUTION

It has been only about a decade since the field of ophthalmology experienced the turning point in its high-tech revolution, a point that will eventually account for the greatest upheaval that this centuries-old medical specialty ever has undergone. Only a few far-thinking physicians were able to recognize it initially, but near the end of the 1970s a number of developments were occurring outside the United States that promised to forever alter the field of ophthalmology for both the patient and the surgeon.

Around that time, more and more U.S. eye surgeons were starting to learn of several exciting experimental programs that were taking place elsewhere. They began to hear about the refractive surgery for nearsightedness that was being performed in Russia by Professor Svyatoslav Fyodorov, and about studies on the more complex technique of keratomeleusis that were being conducted in Colombia by Dr. Jose Barraquer. Additionally, a number of experiments on superior methods of cataract extraction and the implantation of technically superior intraocular lenses (IOLs) also were making headlines in various publications of ophthalmology.

A Good Place To Start

The successful introduction of IOLs may have been the single most important development in today's eye-care revolution, for it showed both physicians and patients that high technology, when properly applied, could dramatically improve their surgical results. Since these lenses offered a new and viable alternative to the postoperative use of contact lenses, however, it is somewhat ironic to note that many of the ophthalmologists who earned their medical degrees during this period actually found that contact lenses were a natural place to begin their new practices.

Due to continuing improvements in contact lenses themselves and a growing perception that they could provide a visual as well as psychological edge for certain patients, more and more Americans were turning to them from standard eyeglasses. Contacts rapidly became the hottest thing in ophthalmology, and many eye doctors who dispensed them soon found their practices booming as a result.

As the number of contact wearers continued to grow, however, so did the number who eventually found that for one reason or another they could not tolerate their lenses. Sometimes their difficulty stemmed from an allergic reaction to the material in the lenses; sometimes it resulted from a job change that placed them suddenly within a dusty, highly polluted environ-ment. For these patients—as well as the ophthalmologists who wanted to help them—surgical procedures designed to correct nearsightedness and farsightedness came along at just the right time.

Surgical Pioneers Pressed On

Even though the preliminary experiments on refractive sur-gery that had taken place in Russia and Colombia were re-ceiving generally positive reviews from knowledgable sources, many American physicians displayed an initial reluctance to recommend and undertake the new procedures. While this un-dercurrent of opposition was bubbling, another group of sur-geons was starting to recognize the great potential of refractive surgery. They realized that to truly help certain patients to the best of their ability, refractive surgery might indeed be the only real answer.

As might be expected, a number of obstacles were en-countered by these surgical pioneers, such as the rejected at-tempts to perform these new procedures at certain hospitals around the country and the negative media reports that were built around a few isolated problems. Eye surgeons who perser-vered often were forced to explain their motives in hostile local newspapers after spending thousands of dollars to purchase their own equipment.

Nonetheless, the satisfaction that came when refractive surgery was finally performed on an appreciative patient quickly negated all of the previous hassles. And so did the op-portunity to work alongside other, innovative eye surgeons who were willing to attempt a series of new and dramatic pro-cedures that they knew would help their patients greatly.

Refractive Controversy Continued

While the simplest of these refractive procedures (Fyodorov's manual technique called radial keratotomy or RK) was gaining a slow but steady acceptance around the country, Barraquer's more radical process (known as keratomeleusis or KM) was stirring up new controversy. Part of the image problem with KM developed because many American surgeons were simply unable to duplicate Barraquer's success, although physicians who support the procedure contend this was generally due to the Americans' unsuccessful attempt to alter a proven procedure to fit their own needs.

Performing a successful KM with the use of a cryolathe turned out to be a real challenge, and today there are only about a dozen eye surgeons in the United States who are accurately utilizing the procedure with a high degree of reproducible results. Those who have invested the time that is necessary to perfect their technique and the $150,000 or so that is necessary to purchase their equipment, however, have discovered what may very well be the best investments they will ever make. Reshaping a patient's cornea—and thus helping to reshape his life—can prove to be the most rewarding process in all of ophthalmology.

Cataract Improvements Are Also Helpful

The recent changes that have come about in cataract surgery, mostly due to the advent of similar high-tech advances, have also proven extremely beneficial to the patient and gratifying to the surgeon. In the past, the diagnosis of a cataract could usually be a very frightening experience that accompanied vivid images of painful surgery, lengthy recovery, and permanently inferior vision. Fortunately, today's techniques and technology have turned all of that completely around.

Again, as recently as the late 1970s, cataract surgery was also a relatively primitive procedure. One basic technique—intracapsular cataract extraction—was used by most surgeons; IOL implantation was still a controversial topic that had both avid supporters and strong detractors. A series of technological revisions during the last few years, however, has shifted most cataract surgeons toward the more successful extracapsular method of extraction. And the vast improvements that have recently been made to intraocular lenses also have guaranteed that their implantation would become standard operating procedure in the truest sense of the term. No longer are either of these high-tech procedures the least bit controversial.

Today, however, cataract surgery has taken another giant leap forward with the advent of phacoemulsification. Even at some of the nation's largest hospitals, only a couple of ophthalmologists are performing this technically demanding operation which requires the highest level of bimanual dexterity. But because of the tiny incision that it requires, as well as the fact that a patient can be virtually assured of excellent sight within one week of surgery, those performing phacoemulsification insist that it offers the most success of any extraction method.

SURGERY IS JUSTIFICATION

For these eye surgeons, particularly, the time that is spent in an operating room is the real justification for entering this very difficult and demanding profession in the first place. They enjoy the periods that are spent in their offices, of course, when they are examining patients and caring for their preoperative and postoperative needs. But it is in the operating room, with a hopeful patient before them and a gallery of high-tech ophthalmic equipment at their fingertips, that it all comes together.

Like an auto mechanic who really enjoys tinkering with cars or an airline pilot who truly enjoys flying a plane, many ophthalmologists savor the time they spend in surgery. They say they find that the apparent tension of the operating room actually provides them with a relaxing and peaceful situation, and that, if it were at all possible, they would prefer to be there for all of their working hours.

Not all eye surgeons are like this, of course, and some really do not enjoy their time in the operating room. These ophthalmologists are terribly nervous about the outcome, they fret about the results, and their uncertainty will occasionally lead them to mistakes. Unfortunately, they are often in the profession only for the money it can bring them and would be the

first to leave if they could find something else that was as finan-
cially rewarding.

Those who love their work, however, are the ones who are
loved by their patients as well as their support staff. They are the
ones who welcome the new tools and techniques that will allow
their patients to see better and then pursue new careers and
lifestyles. And they are the ones who are in awe of the eye itself,
the marvelously intricate organ that has provided centuries of
wondrous speculation for scientist and layman alike. These eye
surgeons, in fact, would probably have had to invent the specialty for themselves if it already did not exist.

OPHTHALMOLOGY *IS* DIFFERENT

The study and correction of an eye problem is actually
quite different from similar work that is performed on something
like the abdomen, which really cannot be viewed without a
great deal of surgical advance work. As the body's only visible
organ, everything about the eye is right up front and obvious to
the trained observer. A surgeon can look into it and see everything that has been done to it previously. The first examination
by an ophthalmologist will yield the entire history of any eye.
Nothing can escape.

Perhaps it is at least partly because of this very obvious nature that ophthalmic researchers are continually driven on to
newer and greater heights. The eye and any problems that be-
fall it, after all, cannot easily be ignored and should be immediately confronted. Our society has thus come to demand a
lot from its eye surgeons, and they in turn have tried to meet that
demand.

We know now that many common causes of vision impairment and blindness are preventable or correctable with proper
high-tech treatments. We know now that eye problems that are
associated with aging do not have to cause people to automatically lose their sight as they enter their later years. We
know now that corrective lenses are not the only way to solve
certain visual deficiencies. And we know now that more and

better treatments will be uncovered at a continually ac-
celerated pace.

Caring and far-thinking eye surgeons have brought us to
this point in our ophthalmic history, and they will be the ones
that will carry us even further. Ophthalmic developments continue to progress at a mind-boggling pace and it is up to the
eye surgeons of the present and the eye surgeons of the future
to guide us toward these ever-changing new horizons that we
call "future vision."

While it is impossible to predict precisely where tomorrow's
still-evolving advances will take us, we can be sure of at least
one thing. The world of eye care will continue to offer an exciting journey—for patient and physician alike.

Further Resources

Those interested in obtaining more information on any of the procedures described in *Future Vision,* as well as those seeking an ophthalmologist to perform them, can find assistance through a number of national and local organizations. Listed below are a variety of groups that can help in either of these searches.

NATIONAL ORGANIZATIONS

American Academy of Ophthalmology, P.O. Box 7424, San Francisco, CA 94120.

American Association for Pediatric Ophthalmology and Strabismus, 800 Westwood Plaza, Suite B, Los Angeles, CA 90024.

American Intra-Ocular Implant Society, 5600 West Addison Street, Chicago, IL 60634.

American Ophthalmological Society, 200 First Street SW, Rochester, MN 55905.

American Society of Contemporary Ophthalmology, 211 East Chicago Avenue, Suite 1044, Chicago, IL 60611.

American Society of Ophthalmic Plastic and Reconstructive Surgery, 1300 North Vermont Avenue, Suite 904, Los Angeles, CA 90027.

Contact Lens Association of Ophthalmology, 2620 Jena Street, New Orleans, LA 70115.

Kerato-Refractive Society, P.O. Box 145, Dennison, TX 75020.

Pan-American Association of Ophthalmology, 150 Shoreline Highway, Building D, Suite 1, Mill Valley, CA 94941.

Macula Society, Department of Ophthalmology, University Hospitals, Iowa City, IA 52242.

National Eye Institute, 9000 Rockville Pike, Building 31, Room 6A03, Bethesda, MD 20205.

Ocular Microbiology and Immunology, Baylor College of Medicine, 6501 Fannin, Houston, TX 77030.

Outpatient Ophthalmic Surgery Society, 1920 116th Avenue NE, Bellevue, WA 98004.

Retina Society, 100 Charles River Plaza, Boston, MA 02114.

LOCAL ORGANIZATIONS

Alabama Academy of Ophthalmology, P.O. Box 11252, Birmingham, AL 35202.

Alaska State Ophthalmological Society, Box 1629, Soldotna, AK 99669.

Arizona Ophthalmological Society, 221 East Camelback Road, Suite 1, Phoenix, AZ 85012.

Arkansas Ophthalmological Society, 45 Pine Manor Drive, Little Rock, AR 72207.

California Association of Ophthalmology, 2655 Van Ness Avenue, San Francisco, CA 94109.

Colorado Ophthalmological Society, P.O. Box 4834, Englewood, CO 80155.

Connecticut Society of Eye Physicians, P.O. Box 30, Bloomfield, CT 06002.

Delaware Academy of Ophthalmology, 1925 Lovering Avenue, Wilmington, DE 19806.

District of Columbia Medical Society/Section on Ophthalmology, 2007 Eye Street NW, Washington, DC 20006.

Florida Society of Ophthalmology, 2020 West Fairbanks Avenue, Winter Park, FL 32789.

Georgia Society of Ophthalmology, 938 Peachtree Street NE, Atlanta, GA 30309.

Hawaii Ophthalmological Society, Kapiolani Children's Medical Center, 1319 Punahou Street, Suite 1110, Honolulu, HI 96826.

Idaho Society of Ophthalmology, 407 West Bannock Street, P.O. Box 2668, Boise, ID 83701.

Illinois Association of Ophthalmology, 20 North Michigan Avenue, Suite 700, Chicago, IL 60602.

Indiana Academy of Ophthalmology, 1820 Alta Vista Street, Munster, IN 46321.

Iowa Academy of Ophthalmology, RR #1, Carlisle, IA 50047.

Kansas Medical Society/Section on Ophthalmology, P.O. Box 8253, Wichita, KS 62708.

Kentucky Academy of Eye Physicians and Surgeons, 301 Muhammad Ali Boulevard, Louisville, KY 40202.

Louisiana Ophthalmological Association, 4116 Jackson Street, Alexandria, LA 71301.

Maine Society of Eye Physicians and Surgeons, 524 Western Avenue, Augusta, ME 04330.

Maryland Society of Eye Physicians and Surgeons, 7901 Annapolis Road, Suite 203, Lanham, MD 20706.

Massachusetts Society of Eye Physicians and Surgeons, P.O. Box 128, Brighton, MA 02135.

Michigan Ophthalmological Society, 302 Eastland Professional Building, Harper Woods, MI 48225.

Minnesota Academy of Ophthalmology, 7600 Parklawn Avenue, Suite 268, Minneapolis, MN 55435.

Mississippi Eye, Ear, Nose, and Throat Association, P.O. Box 12314, Jackson, MS 39211.

Missouri Ophthalmological Society, P.O. Box 1028, Jefferson City, MO 65102.

Montana Academy of Ophthalmology, 2021 Eleventh Avenue, Helena, MT 59601.

Nebraska Academy of Ophthalmology, 1512 First National Bank Building, Lincoln, NE 68508.

Nevada Ophthalmological Society, Suite 530, 3006 South Maryland Parkway, Las Vegas, NV 89109.

Nevada—Las Vegas Ophthalmological Society, 2200 South Rancho Drive, Suite 122, Las Vegas, NV 89102.

New Hampshire Society of Eye Physicians and Surgeons, 5 Coliseum Avenue, Nashua, NH 03060.

New Jersey Academy of Ophthalmology and Otolaryngology, 15 South 9th Street, Newark, NJ 07107.

New Mexico Society of Ophthalmology, 465 St. Michael's Drive, Suite 114, Santa Fe, NM 87501.

New York State Ophthalmological Society, 210 Clinton Road, New Hartford, NY 13413.

North Carolina Society of Ophthalmology, 222 North Person Street, P.O. Box J Box 27167, Raleigh, NC 27611.

North Dakota Academy of Ophthalmology and Otolaryngology, 810 East Rosser, Bismark, ND 58501.

Ohio Ophthalmological Society, 600 South High Street, Columbus, OH 43215.

Oklahoma State Society of Ophthalmology, 5500 North Lincoln, Oklahoma City, OK 73105.

Oregon Academy of Ophthalmology, P.O. Box 13085, Salem, OR 97305.

Pennsylvania Academy of Ophthalmology and Otolaryngology, P.O. Box 1325, Reading, PA 19603.

Puerto Rico Ophthalmological Society, Tulipan #190, San Francisco, Rio Piedras, PR 00927.

Rhode Island Ophthalmological Society, 6 Bedford Road, Pawtucket, RI 02860.

South Carolina Society of Ophthalmology, P.O. Box 11188, Columbia, SC 29211.

South Dakota Academy of Ophthalmology, 2800 Third Street, Rapid City, SD 57701.

Tennessee Academy of Ophthalmology, 112 Louise Avenue, Nashville, TN 37203.

Texas Ophthalmological Association, 1801 North Lamar Boulevard, Austin, TX 78701.

Utah Ophthalmological Society, 540 East Fifth South, Salt Lake City, UT 84102.

Vermont Ophthalmological Society, 1 South Prospect Street, Burlington, VT 05401.

Virginia Society of Ophthalmology and Otolaryngology, 4205 Dover Road, Richmond, VA 23221.

Washington State Academy of Ophthalmology, 900 South Capitol Way, Olympia, WA 98501.

West Virginia Academy of Ophthalmology, P.O. Box 7395, Huntington, WV 25776.

State Medical Society of Wisconsin/Section on Ophthalmology, 850 Elm Grove Road, Elm Grove, WI 53122.

Wyoming Ophthalmology Society, P.O. Drawer 4009, Cheyenne, WY 82003.

Glossary

Acuity: See **Visual Acuity**.

Aphakic: An eye without its normal crystalline lens

Argon laser: An ophthalmic laser that can be used to surgically treat such eye ailments as glaucoma and retinal detachment

A-Scan: A test which measures the eye's length by means of sound waves or ultrasound prior to cataract surgery so that the ophthalmologist can calculate the strength of an intraocular lens to be implanted

Astigmatism: One of the three common refractive errors, which is caused by an unequal curvature present in the shape of the eye's cornea

Aqueous humor: The liquid that occupies the space between the crystalline lens and the cornea

Bifocal: A corrective lens with two different prescriptions, one for near vision and one for distant vision

Binocular indirect ophthalmoscope: A headband-mounted device that allows the ophthalmologist to examine the patient's retina through all but the densest of cataracts

B-Scan: A method of examining the retina when cataracts prevent its viewing by the more commonly used binocular indirect ophthalmoscope

Capsule: One of the three parts that make up the eye's crystalline lens; it is a clear membrane that encases the other two—the nucleus and the cortex

Cataract: A commonly occuring eye ailment, especially among the elderly, in which the crystalline lens becomes cloudy and vision becomes impaired

Cataract spectacles: Heavy "bottle" glasses that, until about thirty years ago, were the only way for postoperative cataract patients to regain visual acuity

Choroid: The membrane adjoining the retina, which, if caused to disconnect, results in a retinal detachment

Concave lens: A corrective lens used to compensate for myopia; it is thicker at the edge than at the center and therefore spreads light rays further apart

Cones and Rods: See **Rods and Cones**.

Conjunctiva: The thin, clear tissue covering the insides of the eyelids and the sclera

Contact lens: A tiny, transparent corrective lens that is placed direclty upon the eye to compensate for refractive errors

Convex lens: A corrective lens used to compensate for hyperopia and presbyopia; it is thicker at the center than at the edge and therefore brings light rays closer together

Cornea: The clear, so-called "window of the eye" that covers the iris and the pupil

Corrective lenses: Prescription eyeglasses or contact lenses that are used to compensate for any of the various refractive errors

Cortex: The soft portion surrounding the nucleus of a crystalline lens that has developed a cataract

Cryoprobe: An ophthalmic instrument that is used in intracapsular cataract extractions to remove a whole cataract from its position within the eye

Cryolathe: An ophthalmic instrument that is used to freeze and reshape a piece of the patient's cornea during a myopic keratomileusis or a hyperopic keratomileusis operation

Crystalline lens: A clear body situated behind the iris that assists in focusing light rays upon the retina

Diamond knife: A precise surgical instrument used in radial keratotomy

Endothelial cell count: An examination that permits the surgeon to determine the health of the patient's cornea and assess its ability to withstand cataract surgery

Epikeratophakia: A form of refractive surgery for extreme cases of myopia and hyperopia in which an ophthalmologist actually sews an additional level of new tissue directly onto the patient's cornea

Extended-wear contact lenses: A relatively new type of contact lens that can be kept in the eye for as long as several weeks at a time

Extracapsular cataract extraction: Currently the most common type of operation for cataract extraction, it involves the separate removal of all of a cataract's individual parts, except for the posterior capsule, which is intentionally left in place

Farsightedness: See **Hyperopia.**

Flashes and floaters: Two common visual symptoms related to the onset of a retinal tear, possibly leading to a retinal detachment

Fluorescein: A solution that is used during certain eye examinations to determine the presence of a number of ailments

Fovea: A portion of the retina that provides acute vision

General anesthetic: A substance that produces a loss of physical sensation as well as a loss of consciousness

Glaucoma: A related group of eye diseases characterized by an increase in the eye's intraocular pressure that, if left untreated, can result in irreversible blindness

Haloes: A colorful ring that appears to encircle various light sources at night and may indicate the presence of cataracts

Hard contact lenses: The first type of contact lens to become publically available and popular

Hyperopia: A refractive error, commonly called *farsightedness,* in which the eye is shorter than normal and therefore prevents proper focusing on nearby objects

Hyperopic keratomeleusis: Also called **HKM,** it is a complicated procedure that utilizes a cryolathe to surgically correct certain cases of hyperopia.

Intracapsular cataract extraction: Until recently the most common form of cataract extraction in the world, it involves the removal of the patient's entire cataract in one piece

Intraocular: Relating to the eye's interior

Intraocular lenses: Permanent replacements for the eye's crystalline lens (called **IOLs** for short) that are usually implanted directly following cataract surgery or at any time thereafter

Intraocular pressure: The force, called **IOP** for short, that is exerted outward by one of two liquids that occurs naturally within the eye

Iridectomy: The surgical removal of a small piece of the iris during cataract surgery to minimize the chances for future development of glaucoma

Iridotomy: See **Iridectomy**.

Iris: The colored portion of the eye that can dilate or constrict to control the amount of light that enters

Keratometry: A test that measures the curvature of the cornea; for example, prior to cataract surgery so that the ophthalmologist can calculate the strength of an intraocular lens to be implanted

Krypton laser: An ophthalmic laser that can be used to surgically treat the abnormal blood vessels that are present in such eye diseases as macular degeneration

Lacrima: The eye's tears or the portion of the eyes that produce or drain these tears

Lasers: see **ophthalmic lasers.**

Lid speculum: A device that is used during eye surgery to keep the patient's eyelids separated

Local anesthetic: A substance that produces a loss of physical sensation without a loss of consciousness

Macular degeneration: Most frequently found among the elderly, it is an eye disease marked by small hemorrhages in the retina that can lead to diminished central or reading vision

Microkeratome: A device used to remove a portion of the patient's cornea during a myopic keratomileusis or a hyperopic keratomileusis procedure

Myopia: A refractive error, commonly called *nearsightedness,* in which the eye is longer than normal and therefore prevents proper focusing on distant objects

Myopic keratomileusis: Also called **MKM,** it is a complicated procedure that utilizes a cryolathe to surgically correct certain cases of myopia

Nearsightedness: See **Myopia.**

Nucleus: The hard central portion, surrounded by the cortex, of a crystalline lens that has developed a cataract

Ocular: Relating to the eye

Operating microscope: The internally lighted, magnifying instrument that allows an ophthalmologist to obtain an accurate and closeup view of his patient's eyes during surgery

Ophthalmic lasers: The ultimate high-tech tools for eye surgery, they are actually a series of slightly different devices that allow the surgeon to accurately and precisely cut tissue and treat diseases of the retina and glaucoma

Ophthalmologist: A medical doctor (MD or osteopath) and surgeon who is specially trained to diagnose and treat diseases and defects of the eye

Ophthalmology: The branch of medical science that is concerned with the structure, functions, and diseases of the eye

Ophthalmoscope: A hand-held instrument that allows the ophthalmologist to examine the patient's retina and optic nerve, unless a cataract is present

Optician: A professional—but not a medical doctor—who is trained to grind and fit the corrective lenses that have been prescribed by an ophthalmologist or an optometrist

Optics: The physical science that deals with light

Optic nerve: A critical part of the eye that transmits visual messages from the retina to the brain

Optometrist: An OD—a Doctor of Optometry but not a medical doctor—who is trained to examine and measure eyes for defects of vision, to prescribe corrective lenses, and to grind and fit these lenses

Outpatient surgery: A modern alternative to automatic overnight hospitalization, which was a standard operating procedure for many years, that allows many surgical patients to return home on the same day that they have undergone a specific operation

Pachymeter: A computerized instrument that helps an eye surgeon determine the depth and placement of radial keratotomy incisions by measuring the thickness of the patient's cornea

Peripheral vision: The area of sight that is outside one's central or reading vision

Phacoemulsification: An advanced form of extracapsular cataract extraction that uses a high-tech tool to break up and remove the cataract's nucleus

Phakic: An eye with its normal crystalline lens

Potential acuity meter: A device, often called a **PAM,** that is mounted on the slit lamp and permits an ophthalmologist to determine whether the patient's poor vision is caused by cataracts or macular degeneration.

Presbyopia: A common defect, related to aging, in which the eye's crystalline lens loses its flexibility and hardens, thus causing an increasing inability to focus properly on nearby objects

Pupil: The dark central portion of the eye through which light enters

Radial keratotomy: A surgical alternative to certain cases of myopia that, for many patients, can eliminate the need for corrective lenses

Refraction: The act of bending light rays that enter the eye so that an image can ultimately be formed on the retina and transmitted to the brain along the optic nerve

Refractive errors: Three commonly occuring visual imper-fections—myopia, hyperopia, and astigmatism—that pre-vent the eye from bending incoming light rays properly

Retina: The final portion of the eye to focus light rays before they are transmitted to the brain along the optic nerve

Retinal detachment: A major cause of blindness that results when the retina separates from its adjoining layer, the choroid

Retinopathy: A major cause of blindness, often the result of di-abetes or hypertension, that generally results from a break-down in the structure, chemistry, or circulation of the retina

Rods and Cones: A group of more than 130 million light-sensitive cells at the back of the retina; rods are for black-and- white vision, cones are for color and daylight vision

Sclera: The white portion of the eye

Slit lamp: An ophthalmic device that is used during most eye examinations so that an ophthalmologist can take a magnified look at the patient's cornea, iris, and crystalline lens

Snellen eye chart: A common wall chart that is used to mea-sure visual acuity

Soft contact lens: A type of contact lens that is soft and pli-able and more comfortable to wear than older models of hard contact lenses

Stitches: See **Sutures.**

Strabismus: An imbalance in the six muscles that control eye movement

Sutures: The threadlike material that is used to close surgical incisions

Tonometer: A device that is used to measure the eye's intraocular pressure and thus check for the presence of glaucoma

Trabeculoplasty: Also called a **filtering operation,** this procedure is designed to keep a patient's intraocular pressure within normal limits by surgically creating a new or improved drainage outlet for his aqueous humor

Visual acuity: A measurement of the eye's visual ability, which, when normal, is commonly expressed as 20/20

Vitreous humor: The clear, jellylike substance that fills the eyeball and gives it its shape

YAG laser: An increasingly popular ophthalmic laser that utilizes the crystal of an yttrium aluminum garnet to create tiny, accurate incisions

About the Authors

ROBERT H. RUBMAN, M.D. was educated at Yale College (A.B.), Massachusetts Institute of Technology (M.S.) and New York University School of Medicine (M.D.), and he pursued research at Harvard Medical School. A Diplomate of the American Board of Ophthalmology, he is currently in private practice at 718 Park Avenue, New York City, and is affiliated with the Manhattan Eye, Ear and Throat Hospital (where he completed his ophthalmology residency), Mt. Sinai Hospital, and Palisade General Hospital. Dr. Rubman has studied intraocular lens implantation, phacoemulsification, neodymium-YAG laser surgery, and keratomileusis and is certified to perform these procedures. He is also cofounder and codirector of the Surgical Eye Institute of New Jersey.

HOWARD ROTHMAN is a journalism graduate from Pennsylvania State University who worked as a reporter and editor on newspapers in three states before becoming a full-time freelance writer in 1983. He specializes in the topics of health and fitness, and his work has appeared in more than forty regional and national publications including *Nation's Business, Home Health Journal, Kiwanis Magazine, Continental Magazine,* and *Denver Business Magazine.* Mr. Rothman currently lives in Denver, Colorado, with his wife and daughter.

Index